CONTROVERSIAL ISSUES IN A DISABLING SOCIETY

21

Disability, Human Rights and Society
Series Editor: Professor Len Barton, Institute of Education, University of London

The *Disability, Human Rights and Society* series reflects a commitment to a particular view of 'disability' and a desire to make this view accessible to a wider audience. The series approach defines 'disability' as a form of oppression and identifies the ways in which disabled people are marginalized, restricted and experience discrimination. The fundamental issue is not one of an individual's inabilities or limitations, but rather a hostile and unadaptive society.

Authors in this series are united in the belief that the question of disability must be set within an equal opportunities framework. The series gives priority to the examination and critique of those factors that are unacceptable, offensive and in need of change. It also recognizes that any attempt to redirect resources in order to provide opportunities for discriminated people cannot pretend to be apolitical. Finally, it raises the urgent task of establishing links with other marginalized groups in an attempt to engage in a common struggle. The issue of disability needs to be given equal significance to those of race, gender and age in equal opportunities policies. This series provides support for such a task.

Anyone interested in contributing to the series is invited to approach the Series Editor at the Institute of Education, University of London.

Current and forthcoming titles

F. Armstrong and L. Barton (eds): *Disability, Human Rights and Education*
P. Beresford: *Psychiatric System Survivors*
M. Corker: *Deaf and Disabled, or Deafness Disabled? Towards a Human Rights Perspective*
M. Corker and S. French (eds): *Disability Discourse*
D. Goodley: *Self-advocacy in the Lives of People with Learning Difficulties*
M. Moore, S. Beazley and J. Maelzer: *Researching Disability Issues*
J. Read: *Disability, the Family and Society: Listening to Mothers*
A. Roulstone: *Enabling Technology: Disabled People, Work and New Technology*
J. Swain, S. French and C. Cameron: *Controversial Issues in a Disabling Society*
C. Thomas: *Female Forms: Experiencing and Understanding Disability*
A. Vlachou: *Struggles for Inclusive Education: An Ethnographic Study*

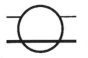

CONTROVERSIAL ISSUES IN
A DISABLING SOCIETY

John Swain

Sally French

Colin Cameron

Open University Press

Open University Press
McGraw-Hill Education
McGraw-Hill House
Shoppenhangers Road
Maidenhead
Berkshire
SL6 2QL
United Kingdom

Email: enquiries@openup.co.uk
World wide web: www.openup.co.uk

and
Two Penn Plaza
New York, NY 10121-2289, USA

First Published 2003
Reprinted 2005

A catalogue record of this book is available from the British Library

ISBN 0 335 20904 1 (pb)   0 335 20905 X (hb)

Library of Congress Cataloging-in-Publication Data
Swain, John
    Controversial issues in a disabling society/John Swain, Sally French and Colin
    Cameron.
       p. cm. – (Disbility, human rights, and society)
    Includes bibliographical references and index.
    ISBN 0-335-20905-X – ISBN 0-335-20904-1 (pbk.)
    1. People with disabilities. 2. People with disabilities – Civil rights.
   3. Discrimination against people with disabilities. 4. Social work with people
   with disabilities. 5. Sociology of disabilities. I. French, Sally. II. Cameron,
   Colin. III. Title. IV. Series.
   HV1568.S93 2003
   362.4–dc21
                                            2002030370

Typeset by Type Study, Scarborough
Printed and bound in Great Britain by Biddles Ltd, King's Lynn, Norfolk

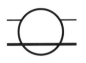

Contents

Series editor's preface

The Disability, Human Rights and Society series reflects a commitment to a social model of disability and a desire to make this view accessible to a wide audience. 'Disability' is viewed as a form of oppression and the fundamental issue is not one of an individual's inabilities or limitations, but rather, a hostile and unadaptive society.

Priority is given to identifying and challenging those barriers to change, including the urgent task of establishing links with other marginalized groups and thus seeking to make connections between class, gender, race, age and disability factors.

The series aims to further establish disability as a serious topic of study, one in which the latest research findings and ideas can be seriously engaged with.

This book is a very welcome addition to the series confirming the centrality of the question of disability as a major means of social differentiation in contemporary society. The book is based on a clear commitment on the part of the authors to the social model of disability in which the disabling nature of society in its varied forms is the focus of careful critical identification and challenge. It is a dynamic conception that is offered in which key assumptions and interpretations are subject to re-examination, providing a more informed knowledge and understanding of fundamental issues as well as a range of ideas and important questions.

In each chapter the authors have carefully contextualized the issue under examination within a more general discussion of relevant concerns, drawing on aspects of appropriate literature, culminating in a case study in which key ideas are perceptively explored and illustrated. A series of questions are also provided that can be used for both personal and group reflection and debates as well as some additional readings to follow up.

The book is very readable, carefully organized and offers a wealth of insights, knowledge and thought-provoking material in which the complexity and contentious nature of the topics are dealt with in imaginative and interesting ways. Existing ideas are critically examined and conceptual, political and pragmatic implications are highlighted. The reader is provided with a clear sense of the seriousness and urgency with which the authors view these issues and their desire that readers do the same.

One of the advantages of this book is that it can be used as a resource in which the wealth of ideas and references can be continually drawn on. The authors have given prominence to the voices of disabled people in such a way that difference is celebrated in a dignified and stimulating manner. It is a challenging read, one which both disturbs and encourages, offers a rich series of insights, ideas and questions in need of further exploration and debate.

Change is of central importance to the authors and overall the book is comprehensive in its coverage of the chosen issues it examines. The concern is to make connections between biographical, situational factors and experiences and global, structural, political conditions and relations. Understanding the world is part of a more general desire for the realization of a truly inclusive society, one in which all disabling, discriminatory and exclusionary assumptions and practices are removed.

This book will hopefully make some contribution to realizing this at both a personal and more collective level.

Len Barton
Institute of Education
London

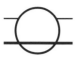

Acknowledgements

Dr Maureen Gillman (case study for Chapter 1); Professor Bob Heyman (case study for Chapter 1); Jack Osborn (case study for Chapter 2); Year 2 (2001–02) Disability Studies Students, University of Northumbria (case study for Chapter 3); Colin Goble (author Chapter 4); Joanna (case study for Chapter 4); Ayesha Vernon (co-author Chapter 5); DASh (Disability Arts in Shropshire), Ruth Kate of DASh (case study for Chapter 6); Connect, Sally Byng of Connect (case study for Chapter 8); Paula Greenwell (co-author Chapter 9); Tina Cook (co-author Chapter 10); Joan Adams (co-author Chapter 11); Southampton Centre for Independent Living (case study for Chapter 12); MK SUN (case study for Chapter 13); Rachel Hurst (author Conclusion).

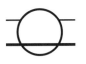

Notes on contributors

Joan Adams, Principle Lecturer, Faculty of Health, Social Work and Education, University of Northumbria.

Colin Cameron, disabled rights activist and Disability Equality Trainer, Leeds.

Tina Cook, Senior Lecturer, Faculty of Health, Social Work and Education, University of Northumbria.

Dr Sally French, Senior Lecturer, King Alfred's College of Higher Education, Winchester and Associate Lecturer, The Open University.

Colin Goble, Senior Lecturer in Learning Disabilities Nursing, School of Health and Social Care, University of Greenwich and doctoral student, School of Health Science, University of Wales, Swansea.

Paul Greenwell, disabled right activist, co-chair Disability Action North East.

Rachel Hurst, disabled rights activist, director of Disability Awareness in Action.

John Swain, Professor of Disability and Inclusion, Faculty of Health, Social Work and Education, University of Northumbria.

Dr Ayesha Vernon, disabled rights activist and Disability Equality Trainer, Leeds.

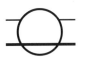

Introduction: enabling questions

What is this book about?

Disability studies is a burgeoning domain of study, as is evident in the growth of courses, research and literature. It has its roots in the growth of the disabled people's movement within Britain and internationally, and the foundation of the social model of disability. Disability studies is centrally the study of the disabling society. At its best it is an arena of critical debate addressing controversial issues concerning, not just the meaning of disability, but the nature of society, dominant values, quality of life, and even the right to live. We begin by considering the rationale by which we deem issues 'controversial'.

The starting point has to be definitions of 'disability' (and related terms). The dominant view of disability is individual or essentialist, that is as something wrong with the individual. A disabled person is thought of as someone who cannot see, cannot hear, cannot walk, has Down syndrome, has a mental illness and so on. The words 'cannot' and 'has' are crucial. What is at fault is the individual and what needs changing is the individual. There has, however, been what is sometimes referred to as a 'paradigm shift', at least for some disabled people. This is a shift in thinking of disability as a condition of the individual, to understanding disability as a condition of a society in which people with impairments are discriminated against, segregated and denied full participative citizenship. It is a shift from 'disabled' being seen as a personal tragedy, to 'disabled' being a positive identity. And it is a shift from dependency and passivity, to the rights of disabled people to control decision-making processes that shape their lives.

As challenges to ways of viewing women came from women themselves (with the feminist movement) and challenges to ways of viewing Black people came from Black people themselves, so challenges to ways of viewing disability have emerged from the disabled people's movement. Disabled people have generated an alternative view: the social model of disability.

From this viewpoint, society is at fault, that is a disabling society that is geared to, built for and by, and controlled by non-disabled people – a society that excludes disabled people. This exclusion is created and constructed in every aspect of living, including ways of thinking, language, the built environment, power structures, information, values, rules and regulations. Whether you are disabled or not you are living in a disabling society. The roots of controversial issues lie in the challenge of individual models by the social model, and there is evidence that, though it is slow, progress is being made. Barnes and Mercer (2001a: 11) state: 'Many people across the world, including politicians and policy makers, now recognize that "disability" is an equal opportunities/human rights issue on a par with sexism, heterosexism, racism and other forms of social exclusion.'

At another level the social model is of itself challenging. There are controversial issues in understanding the social world through the social model. Key concepts are widely deployed and employed in discussions generated by the social model, principally: barriers, discrimination (and institutional discrimination) and oppression. What is the meaning of each of these terms and how do they relate to each other? There are, for instance, different models of barriers. The SEAwall model (Swain et al. 1998) presents one way of conceiving the institutional barriers that prevent people with impairments achieving access to and participation in organizations. Figure 1 depicts these barriers as the bricks in a wall of institutional discrimination. The wall (rather than more usual concentric circles) graphically illustrates the marginalization of disabled people. In this model of institutional discrimination, attitudinal barriers are constructed on environmental barriers, which are themselves constructed on structural barriers. No graphics can depict the interlinking and interaction among the three levels, though ideology plays a key role in the articulation and inter-reliance between each layer. Middleton (1999: 71), however, suggests that this particular model 'is limited in being two dimensional and undynamic, suggesting that any progress is dependent on the whole wall being dismantled at some point in time.' She describes the SEAwall model as 'revolutionary' and contrasts it with other more 'persuasive' models of social change.

This takes the debates into a broader arena that can, as ever, be couched in a number of ways. Essentially, to address disability is to address the nature of the society in which we live as the social, cultural and historical context of disability. We do not live, however, in a society that is solely disablist in oppressing people. Racism, sexism, classism, homophobia and ageism have all generated analyses of the social world. How, for instance, does the social model of disability relate to feminist theories?

To complicate matters further, the social model is not an ossified way of thinking. It is itself the subject of debate and development. Two crucial and often explicitly related arenas of debate are over the capacity of the social model to encompass the personal experiences of all people with impairments and to provide a basis for understanding and studying impairments as well as disability.

Attitudinal

| Cognitive prejudice: assumptions about the (in)abilities, emotional responses, needs of disabled people | Emotional prejudice: fear | Behavioural prejudice: individual practice and praxis |

Environmental

| Disablist language | Institutional policies, organization, rules and regulations | Professional practices: assessment, care management | Inaccessible physical environments |

Structural

| Hierarchical power relations and structures: disempowerment of disabled people | The denial of human, social and welfare rights | Structural inequalities: poverty |

Cemented by ideologies of 'normality' and 'independence'

Figure 1 The SEAwall of institutional discrimination

Disability studies is itself the subject of controversy, in terms of its theoretical basis and who controls courses and research and whether it should be shaped and controlled by disabled academics or grassroots activists or non-disabled academics. There are fundamental challenges to policy, provision and professional practice that are directly relevant to all who work with disabled people, whether in the field of social work, health or education. Again key concepts are the focus of controversy. At the time of writing 'inclusion' has become the catchword in the development of policy, service provision and professional practice and in its wake the questions multiply. How is inclusion different from integration? How is inclusion in policy realized in professional practice? Who controls the decision-making processes in moves towards inclusion?

Finally in this brief overview of our conception of controversial issues in a disabling society, there are the broadest implications of the social model of disability. While the model may underpin academic study and understanding, the social model of disability is essentially about social change. The debates around controversial issues have an ultimate political purpose: to challenge and break down the barriers, discrimination and oppression disabled people face. In this sense, the social model of disability is the vision of the liberation and emancipation of disabled people, through developing collective and individual 'critical consciousness' (McLaren and Leonard 1993) and activation. Debate engendered by controversial issues in a disabling society is not for the sake of debate. It is to change the lives of disabled people, through changing the disabling environment, prejudicial attitudes, and unequal power relations that disable people with impairments and exclude them from full participatory citizenship.

Who is this book for?

This book is aimed at a wide readership including disabled people, professionals and policy makers who are involved with disabled people, whether they themselves are disabled or non-disabled, for example health workers, social workers, teachers and students of these professions. The book will also be of use to academics and students who are teaching or studying disability studies, sociology and 'equality studies' and non-professionals who are involved with disabled people, for example personal assistants and parents. We also hope there will be a wider audience for the book as issues of disability have relevance to us all and a non-disablist society would be better for everyone.

What is in this book?

The book aims to generate questioning and to promote debate. It has three parts. In Part One, we reflect on **Foundations** for the study of disability. These foundations lie in ways of thinking about disability, the language that is used and the struggle for the control of meanings. They include questions about disability studies as a field of study. Disability studies is a relatively new area of academic inquiry which is interdisciplinary and diverse, drawing on psychology, sociology, linguistics, economics, anthropology, politics, history and media studies – but what will it do for disabled people?

Part Two examines **Values and ideologies** that impinge on the day-to-day lives of disabled people. It starts with questions of life and death and the highly controversial notion that life can be unworthy of life. Recent developments in genetics, the human genome project, have served to bring these issues to the fore. There are questions of diverse identities and experiences, depending on ethnic origin, gender, age and other social divisions. Disabled people also challenge dominant values. What's so good about independence? Why is disability seen as a tragedy? Who wants charity? Finally there are questions concerning 'whose body?' There is controversy around the use of cosmetic surgery with people with Down syndrome, cochlear implants for deaf children, and the rights of all disabled people to participate in sexual activity.

Part Three turns to questions of **Policy, provision and practice**. Language and developments that can appear just, progressive and even liberating, are not always what they seem. Changing policy, provision and practice under flags such as meeting special needs, community care and inclusion require close scrutiny in terms of the actual changes in the daily lives of disabled people. The concept of 'needs', for instance, has played a key role in the unequal power relationship between professionals and disabled people, needs being defined and assessed by professionals in controlling the provision of services. Have recent changes in social policy, such as 'direct payments' and a market orientation to health and social care, moved disabled people away from professional control of their lives? Why are disabled people increasingly rejecting the idea of care and arguing that this has been experienced as oppression and control? How can 'carers' be part of the solution rather than part of the problem? The politics of change are being played out in an increasingly broad arena, nationally and internationally. Why have disabled people struggled for civil rights legislation – and why do they continue to do so? Why are disabled people dissatisfied with the Disability Discrimination Act 1995? How far are western ideas about disability relevant to disabled people in the majority world and vice versa?

How to use this book

Controversial Issues in a Disabling Society is not a reader or a straightforward textbook, but rather a resource book of material dealing with specific, substantive issues. It is an introductory book, touching on a wide range of issues. It is a collection of relatively short chapters, each setting questions for discussion, outlining the context of a set of key issues and presenting particular arguments. The book provides a series of analyses that challenge dominant positions and ideologies from a social model viewpoint of disability. The material is designed to lend itself to teaching methods with a high degree of student involvement such as seminars, group discussion and debates.

Each chapter has three sections, working from the most general to the most specific: first, a coverage of general issues; second, an examination of the issues as they apply specifically to disabled people; and third, a case study. The case studies are varied and include the experiences and views of individual disabled people, institutions and organizations. A short list of **Questions for discussion** is provided at the end of each of the three sections of the chapter and a **Debate activity** at the end of the chapter. The aim of the questions is to facilitate you in reflecting on the topics being discussed in the chapter. They are open-ended questions to fuel debate, rather than questions demanding 'right or wrong' answers. There are different types of questions:

1 Some questions ask you to examine the issues in terms of your personal experiences and views. It can be argued that issues are controversial only if they involve you in reflecting on deeply held understandings, values and beliefs.
2 Some questions relate to and can be answered in the context of the discussion in the chapter. These might involve you responding to contrasting views or a particular position that has been presented. We hope that in either case you will take a critical stance to ask your own questions and develop your own arguments.
3 Other questions require you to look beyond the discussion within the chapter. This is an introductory book that we hope will take you beyond our particular arguments. In the questions, and the debate activities, we hope we are raising issues that will give you a basis for exploring the literature, within disability studies and, as relevant, social sciences generally, and also gathering evidence, for instance, from disabled people themselves and their organizations. A short list of 'further reading' is included with each chapter as a starting point.

We hope that the material in this book will help focus and stimulate work in discussion groups, seminars and tutorials. French et al. (1994) state:

> Group discussion is an active, democratic teaching method where each participant has the right to contribute ideas, and in which the teacher does not dominate. The members of the group pool their knowledge and learn from each other. Discussion is a particularly useful method for exploring complex, multifaceted issues. By considering the interpretations and ideas of others, individual learners are provided with a broader perspective.
>
> (French et al. 1994: 86)

Brown and Atkins (1988: 50) warn, however, that 'it is relatively easy to have a vague meandering discussion. It is much more difficult for students to discuss coherently, to question and to think.'

Controversial issues seem to us to have particular use in debates of various kinds. One format we have used follows the steps of Habeshaw et al. (1988).

1 The group is asked to prepare for a tutorial by reading statements that illustrate a variety of viewpoints in a controversial area.
2 At the start of the session the participants are divided into as many subgroups as there are points of view in the controversial area and then each group is asked to prepare a case for its viewpoint. It can be useful to have a proposition for debate, for example: 'we believe that all disabled pupils should be educated in inclusive schools with their non-disabled peers.' The division into subgroups can be random, that is participants are allocated to groups irrespective of their personal beliefs about the issues under discussion. This has the advantage of improving participants' skills in argument and increasing their capacity for understanding the other person's viewpoint. Arguments are less likely to be rejected if counter-arguments are provided.
3 For the debate each subgroup selects a first and second speaker. The first speaker for each subgroup sets out the argument from their viewpoint. After the first speakers, the second speaker from each subgroup attempts to answer points made from the other viewpoints. The debate is then opened up for a free discussion.
4 Finally participants are asked to vote for or against the proposition based on their personal beliefs.

Overall we hope that this book will be of use to you in furthering the debates in the struggle for the liberation and emancipation of all disabled people, changing ways of thinking, breaking down disabling barriers and creating a more inclusive society.

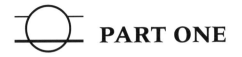 **PART ONE**

FOUNDATIONS

1

What's in a name?

Mind your language

Within a social world the way that we understand the objects and relationships around us are framed within the language that we use. Names are given to objects, groups and categories of phenomena in order to distinguish them from others. This makes it possible for us to understand and control them better and to communicate about them with each other. We begin, then, by examining this process of labelling people and then address the issues in relation to disabled people. The chapter ends with a case study, from research, of labels applied to 'people with learning difficulties'.

The naming and classifying of objects is an activity that has gone on since human beings first evolved. For instance, according to the Bible, God brought 'every beast of the field and fowl of the air to Adam to see what he would call them' (Genesis 2: 19). This naming process signalled the dominion of human beings 'over everything that moves upon the earth' (Genesis 1: 28). When parents choose a name for a newborn child they are placing an identity upon that child. Frequently infants will be given names that come from parents or grandparents in order to establish continuity in lines of genealogy. It is usual for wives to give up their maiden names and to adopt the surnames of their husbands and for children to be given the surnames of their fathers rather than their mothers. This reflects the way in which power is structured within a patriarchal society. As badges of identity the names we are given, or the names we give ourselves, have a powerful influence in shaping our understanding of who we are, where we have come from and where we belong. Designations like 'man/woman', 'black/white', 'old/young', 'Catholic/Protestant', 'gay/straight', 'working class/middle class' are labels by which we come to identify ourselves. They can evoke feelings of superiority or inferiority or be marks of inclusion or exclusion, humiliation or pride. Fundamentally they are reflections of the way in which society is organized and the positions we hold within it. Burr (1997: 7) suggests that language is 'more than simply a way of expressing ourselves. When people talk to each other the world gets constructed. Our use of language can therefore be thought of as a form of social action.'

Labelling is the process whereby descriptions are attached to individuals or groups which, in turn, guides the attitudes and behaviour of others towards them. Labelling theory was first applied to criminal behaviour, where it was noted that the application of labels such as 'criminal' and 'addict' tended to increase the deviant behaviour. One of the reasons for this is that we tend to live up to other people's expectations of us. Labelling somebody negatively may also lead to increased surveillance or segregation from the wider community which further increases (and even creates) the predicted behaviour (Fulcher and Scott 1999). These processes, whereby people tend to live up to the expectations of others, have been termed the self-fulfilling prophecy (Gross 1987).

A major factor in the labelling process is that labels are usually bestowed by those who have power and authority ('experts') upon those who do not. Fiske (1993) referred to this as 'imperialising' power. Power of this type was present in the British colonies where a minority of influential British people controlled indigenous populations by means of force, coercion and western ideologies which were geared towards maintaining control (Potter 2000).

Professionals including doctors, social workers, psychologists and teachers are endorsed with institutional authority to make judgements and impose labels on people. By virtue of the recognized knowledge and qualifications they have gained through education, they are judged to have demonstrated their fitness to make valid pronouncements on the 'cases' with whom they deal. The education that they have received, however, has not taken place in a social vacuum but reflects existing relationships of power within society. Professionals are granted social power only as long as they conform with the codes of practice and values of their professions. The judgements that they make and the labels they impose reflect particular cultural norms. By defining what is considered aberrant the boundaries of what is deemed acceptable (or normal) are marked out (Thomson 1997).

Labelling is not, however, the exclusive domain of the powerful. People may label themselves ('I'm a cockney') and label each other ('he's a Geordie'). Such labels may be positive or negative, enduring or transient. In the 1950s gangs of rebellious young men, who dressed and behaved in a certain way, labelled themselves 'Teddy boys', and in the 1960s two rival groups, the 'mods' and the 'rockers', noted for their motorbikes and physical combat in seaside towns, emerged to enrage the 'respectable' majority. People may be labelled by the school they attended ('he's an old Etonian'), by their sexual orientation ('I'm a dyke'), or by their country or origin ('she's a Yank').

In themselves names are not necessarily good or bad. They can be used either positively or negatively, to affirm a person's identity or to oppress, coerce, control and exclude (Saraga 1998). Naming can, on the one hand, be an exercise of power and part of a process of control but, on the other hand, be an expression of personal or group identity and part of a process of liberation.

Questions for discussion

1 Some labels can be seen as more stigmatizing than others. Think about yourself in terms of labels applied to you. What labels do you accept as positive and aspire to? What labels do you find offensive and demeaning? Why?

2 What positive and negative labels do you give to yourself? How far do these tally with labels given to you by others?

3 Is it possible to resist the labels we are given by others, for example by teachers and parents and acquire new ones? How can we achieve this?

Disabling and enabling labels

The words used to describe disabled people are almost invariably negative or passive. They may, for example, be labelled by their impairment ('he's a paraplegic', 'she's an amputee') as if that were their most important attribute. Many words in common use, for example 'short-sighted', meaning lack of insight, show how deeply rooted negative perceptions of disability are in our culture. The very words 'disabled' (not able) and 'invalid' (not valid) indicate the lowly status that disabled people have within society. Stone (1999a) found similar conceptions of disabled people in her studies of ancient Chinese script.

Descriptions of disabled people frequently have tragic overtones, for example 'sufferers' and 'victims', and they are often spoken of as an homogeneous group, for example 'the disabled' and 'the blind', which is reflected in the titles of many leading charities. Disabled people are also referred to as 'patients' and 'clients' and are thought to have 'needs' rather than 'rights'. As French and Sim (1993: 31) state, 'Basic human rights are often regarded as disabled people's needs, for example the "need" for an accessible toilet.'

Some labels applied to disabled people, such as 'brave' and 'extraordinary' appear, on the surface, to be positive but are regarded by disabled people as negative. This is because such descriptions give a distorted image with which few disabled people can identify. French (1989: 30) states that such words 'either gives rise to the notion that disabled people are superhuman, or that anything they achieve – however minor – is worthy of congratulation and admiration.'

The euphemism 'physically challenged' gives rise to images of disabled people keenly and happily struggling against adversity within a disabling society, while being admired for doing so. It reinforces the notion that society is fixed and that disabled people must 'overcome' what are viewed as 'their' problems if they are ever to become valid members of it.

An issue which gives rise to considerable discussion is whether the term 'disabled people' or 'people with disabilities' should be used. 'People with disabilities' is said to humanize disabled people by putting the person before the disability. It implies that we have only to change our attitudes in order to change the realities around us. Oliver and Barnes (1998), however, draw attention to a number of important negative implications arising from the tendency to place the word 'people' before 'disability'. They point out that it blurs the distinction between impairment and disability implying that disability is the property of disabled people and not society. It sidesteps the need for social and environmental change and explicitly denies the political nature of disability. Placing the word 'disabled' before the word 'people', on the other hand, is a political statement arising from the understanding that disability is 'done' to people rather than being something that they 'have'.

The same tendency to obscure the political meaning of disability can be found in the use of euphemisms aimed, ostensibly, at drawing attention away from people's impairments. In her discussion of the term 'differently abled' for instance, Wendell (1997) states:

> I assume the point of using this term is to suggest that there is nothing wrong with being the way we are, just different. Yet to call someone 'differently abled' is much like calling her 'differently coloured' or 'differently gendered'. . . If anything, it increases the 'otherness' of disabled people, because it reinforces the paradigm of young, strong and healthy, with all body parts working perfectly.
>
> (Wendell 1997: 271–2)

Many people labelled as being learning disabled prefer the term 'people with learning difficulties'. Brechin (1999) explains that this puts the person before the 'problem' which, given their history of extreme segregation, abuse and neglect, may be particularly important. It is also a less all-embracing term than 'mentally handicapped' which preceded it and suggests that people are capable of learning if given the opportunity to do so. Brechin does, however, find the term problematic for the same reasons put forward by Oliver and Barnes (1998) in their discussion of disabled people generally. She states that, 'If the whole problem *by definition* lies *with* the individual, then our understandings and our interventions start and stop with the individual' (Brechin 1999: 58, emphasis in original).

There is, however, considerable controversy about this issue by the recipients of such labels. Aspis, who describes herself as 'a disabled person who has been labelled by the system as having learning difficulties' (1999: 174), says that the name and the identity 'learning difficulties' 'have been imposed upon me by the system, in particular the education system, which pre-defines learning ability' (Aspis 1999: 174). Other people labelled as having learning difficulties reject the process of labelling altogether as the following quotations illustrate:

Nobody has got learning difficulties, everyone is clever.

(French and Swain 1999: 328)

I'm thinking that disabled is not the right word. I'm thinking that you're still a human being that . . . we are put here on this world to be loved and be cared for, not to be called names . . . labelling should be banned completely, right off, and scrub it right in the bin, the scrap heap.

(Palmer et al. 1999: 36)

One of the slogans of People First, an organization of people labelled as having learning difficulties, is Label Jars not People. It is worth mentioning here that many people labelled in this way were deemed ineducable and were given no formal education until a change in the law in 1970. This clearly illustrates how words are translated into policy and practice.

Since the introduction of the term 'special educational needs' in the Warnock Report (1978), the label 'special needs' has gained common currency and has become recognized as a legitimate personal description, for example 'Jimmy has special needs' or 'I'm a special needs teacher'. This may, in turn, lead disabled children to identify and measure themselves as 'other than' or 'less than' supposedly 'normal' children (Middleton 1999). The term 'special educational needs', and the practices that emanate from it, have been criticized for stigmatizing children, for producing a negative, homogenous category, and for being uncritical of educational practice and maintaining the status quo (Armstrong et al. 2000). This sense of stigmatization and difference is clearly evident in the following quotation from a teenage boy with a visual impairment who is talking about his special school, 'I'm not worried about telling them where it is, I'm worried about telling them what it is. I tell them it's a private school' (Swain and French 1998: 98).

As the names used to identify people with impairments reflect dominant discourses of tragedy and inferiority, it is not surprising that many disabled people are unwilling to identify themselves as disabled. A disabled person quoted by Shakespeare et al. (1996: 51), for example, states, 'I was in denial about being disabled most of the time, and if I saw anyone who was disabled I didn't want to talk to them, and if I did talk to them, it was as if I was able-bodied . . . doing the old patronising bit.'

However, although the discourse is usually about the labelling of disabled people by others, disabled people have also labelled themselves and in so doing have turned negative labels into proud labels. People in the Deaf community write 'deaf' with a capital 'D' as a symbol of self-respect, strength and solidarity, and labels such as 'crip' are used by disabled people in a similar way. Marta Russell, the author of *Beyond Ramps* (Russell 1998), for example, describes herself as an 'uppity crip'. Labelling by disabled people themselves celebrates difference and fosters a collective identity. This is what Fiske (1993) terms 'localising power', that is the bottom-up power of subordinated groups.

Questions for discussion

1 What are the implications of labelling for disabled people in terms of
personal and political control over identity and quality of life? What
labels might disabled people accept as positive and aspire to? Why?
2 How successful have disabled people been in naming themselves?
Has this had any implications for policy and practice?
3 Do disabled people need labels?

Questioning labels

This case study is based on research conducted at the University of Northumbria (Swain et al. 1999; Gillman et al. 2000). Two projects explored the processes and meaning of labelling, particularly labels of 'learning difficulties',
'challenging behaviour' and 'autism'. Semi-structured interviews and focus
groups were conducted with people with learning difficulties, family carers,
care workers and professionals, including social workers, general practitioners, psychiatrists and nurses. The research addressed the processes by
which people are labelled and the implications of labels in determining interventions. Here we shall concentrate on the views and experiences of care
workers and family carers.

Challenging behaviour is one of the most problematic labels in terms of
definitions and criteria for labelling, the processes by which people are
labelled and the consequences of being labelled. The most common behaviours thought to be challenging in this research involved some form of
violence or aggression towards staff or other service users. However, a wide
range of behaviours was deemed to be challenging including sexual assault:

> He put his hand upon my breast, and said, 'I'm sick of this place'. I took
> hold of his hand, removed it and said, 'Leave it', or something like that.
> And because I had removed his hand, he sort of nipped us quite badly on
> the arm.

One interesting point about this statement is that such sexual abuse is referred
to as challenging. If this had been an example of abuse perpetrated by, rather
than upon, staff, it would not have been regarded as challenging behaviour.
The next example underlines this point. Here expressions of dislike for a day
centre are seen as challenging:

> We had experience here of a behaviour which was quite challenging, that
> the person concerned would come in, she is from a different cultural
> background, so that had a bearing on it. But she would come in, and
> would wail and scream, and would be totally inconsolable . . . She
> wouldn't even attempt to propel her wheelchair, even though, to all
> intents and purposes she appeared to be capable of doing so, but would
> really drown out any attempt that you had to talk to her.

As in the previous example, similar defiance by staff would not be deemed challenging as such, however unacceptable it was thought to be. Another question arising from this quotation is whether overcompliance would be seen to be as challenging as behaviours that might be said to resist the status quo such as silent acceptance of verbal abuse from other clients or staff.

The consequences of behaviour were also referred to in defining what is challenging, particularly dangers to the person themselves or others:

> I think it is not taken seriously unless there's physical contact, someone actually is violent towards you, or furniture, whatever. The everyday somebody screaming all day, you'd say that is challenging, but it's not taken really seriously unless people are hurt. Something that puts them or others in danger basically seems to be the main criteria.

Perhaps inevitably, one factor in whether behaviour is seen as challenging or not is whether it is manageable, and this depends on a variety of considerations, including predictability:

> The two people I've got, one of them, there's trigger points, you can actually see the signs of him building up. And you know that there's going to be an outburst, for want of a better expression, you know, well, towards you. The other person shows no signs at all. There's no trigger points, nothing, and she can just become very, very violent towards you for no reason at all.

Though the care workers found it easy to identify examples of challenging behaviour and people whose behaviour was seen as challenging, they also talked of the difficulties of defining what is challenging, suggesting, for instance, that such judgements are relative to individual values:

> It depends how people see it as a, you know, what I might see as a challenging behaviour you mightn't.

It seemed, too, that the label of challenging was not just dependent on who was making the judgement but who was being judged. Some behaviours could be acceptable from one person but not another.

The research suggested that labels can be seen in a more positive light. Some participants sought diagnosis and labelling in the belief that they would be followed by treatment, intervention or social support that would lead to a better quality of life for the individual and possibly the family. Expert knowledge is not necessarily the exclusive territory of professionals. Family carers make it their business to access what they consider to be appropriate medical knowledge, which is then incorporated into their explanations about their relatives' symptoms and behaviour. A family carer told us how she had been convinced for many years that her son was 'autistic', a diagnosis that was finally given when her son was in his twenties:

> When Malcolm was growing up, we read articles about autism, and I approached the school. I was told, 'You are always looking for answers, accept that Malcolm has learning difficulties and then you will overcome all of your problems.'

A label can provide an explanation that can be useful to family carers in their dealings with the general public and, indeed, professionals. Misunderstandings of individuals' behaviour can lead to disapproval and assumptions about the person with learning difficulties and his or her family. Two participants commented:

> with the autistic kid we fostered, I used to want a sheet of paper to hand around to people to explain what was going on . . . he looked like a naughty boy who had control over me. This is what it looked like and it's how the public picked it up as well.

The need for a formal label also was seen as important by those carers whose son's or daughter's learning difficulty was not immediately visible:

> I used to wish that he was in a wheelchair or that he had Down's Syndrome, so people could see he was different from other children.

Nevertheless labelling people is a powerful business and raises numerous thorny questions. What are the consequences for the labelled person? Is it a basis for a better understanding or does it invoke stereotyping and discriminatory assumptions about a person's worth which can be used to justify the exclusion of an individual from treatment such as organ transplantation and dialysis. A participant commented:

> If you and I as adults began to develop a continence problem, we would be sent for screening and possible treatment. If you've got learning difficulties and you have developed this in adulthood, it is accepted to be just part of learning difficulties.

The label challenging behaviour can precipitate management procedures. A key worker from a day centre, for instance, described the behavioural programme that had been designed by a clinical psychologist to enable staff to deal with challenging behaviour.

The research suggested, however, that the consequences of labelling can be highly detrimental. A keyworker from a day centre, for instance, described the behavioural programme that had been designed by a clinical psychologist to enable staff to deal with challenging behaviour:

> Once we start having outbursts from her, she'd be directed to the time-out chair. She can use the time-out for up to fifteen minutes . . . If she is calm for up to two minutes, she can leave the chair. If after fifteen minutes she is still being aggressive then we have to bring her into the time-out room, and she is allowed to stay in there for five minutes . . . we hold the door handle just to stop her getting out. After five minutes we can actually lock the door, and that's classed as seclusion . . . When she has these outbursts she's given medication.
>
> (Gillman et al. 1997: 686)

In this instance the purpose of labelling is to instigate control of the person being labelled.

Questions for discussion

1 Are you ever thought to have challenging behaviour? If so, what are these behaviours and what effect do they have on you and other people?
2 Are there any circumstances under which being labelled as a person with challenging behaviour might have positive consequences?
3 The term 'challenging' has certain connotations when applied to the behaviour of people with learning difficulties, all of which are negative and problem related. Why is this?

Debate activity

Debate the proposition: Labelling disabled people is always harmful. The following quotations may provide you with a starting point:

> I'm done with names. Names are nothing but collars men tie around your neck to drag you where they like.
>
> (Gray 2001: 72)

> Discovering that your child has a specific need or disability is probably one of the most devastating experiences that a parent will live through . . . we have information on over 1000 rare syndromes and rare disorders and can put families in touch with each other . . . our definition of children with disabilities includes children who are born with specific and rare disorders, children who develop acute and long-term health conditions and children who have special educational needs.
>
> (Contact a Family 2001)

Further reading

Brechin, A. (1999) Understandings of learning disability, in J. Swain and S. French (eds) *Therapy and Learning Difficulties: Advocacy, Participation and Partnership*. Oxford: Butterworth-Heinemann.

Corker, M. and French, S. (eds) (1999) *Disability Discourse*. Buckingham: Open University Press.

Fulcher, J. and Scott, J. (1999) *Sociology*. Oxford: Oxford University Press.

Saraga, E. (ed.) (1998) *Embodying the Social: Constructions of Difference*. London: Routledge.

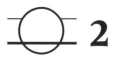 **2**

Whose model?

Ways of thinking about the social world

This chapter begins by considering the ways in which our perceptions and experiences of reality are informed by particular models and frameworks that reflect dominant practices within particular societies and cultures. Bauman (1997) describes culture as a 'purposeful activity' which imposes an artificial order upon social life, calls that order natural, right and desirable, and works to maintain that order at the expense of alternatives which it represents as inferior and disorderly. The discussion then moves to models of disability and ends with a case study of Jack, a man with dyslexia.

Culture is an activity that reflects attempts by human beings to impose certain frameworks upon the ways in which we relate to each other, to establish boundaries between what is right and wrong, acceptable and unacceptable, proper and improper, normal and abnormal. It is a necessary activity; without culture there would be no guidelines for understanding either who we are, where we have come from, what we should do, or where we are going.

However, culture is also a distorting activity. Dominant (or mainstream) cultures will always reflect the interests of those within particular social groups or societies who have the power to define situations and the resources with which to ensure that their own definitions are accepted as true. Those whose interests conflict with those of the powerful are represented, to various extents, as uncivilized, degenerate, immoral, inadequate or incapable (Saraga 1998).

Finally, culture is an activity that harnesses, in its interests, the social institutions that hold a society together. The legal, economic, educational and civil structures by which populations are bound are organized in ways which confirm and give legitimacy to the version of reality that has been sanctioned by those with power. Culture, then, is a process that shapes our expectations and experiences. The culture we grow up in provides the 'coloured glasses' through which we understand our social world and ourselves. Personal identity and the identity of 'others' are grounded within the ways of thinking and doing within that culture.

While each of us may experience our own individuality as being of utmost significance, it should not be overlooked that what distinguishes us from those around us is much less that what connects us. Each of us comes into a world that is not of our own making. The identities that are initially ascribed to us and which we negotiate as we grow and gain experience are structured around a set of variables such as age, class, gender, ethnicity, sexuality, disability and religion (Kalekin-Fishman 2001). While we may experience our own individuality as unique, the range of identities available to us is limited and structured around currently prevailing culturally accepted ideas.

We grow and learn by coming to recognize the people and objects around us and by interacting within a process whereby we establish relationships with our environment and our environment stamps its mark on us. Even if we are to question them later on, we absorb the values, customs, patterns of behaviour, beliefs and traditions of those who are responsible for our protection and guidance. We are told that this is the way the world is and, until we develop a critical consciousness, we tend to accept that this is the way it must be (Friere 1996). This is not particularly controversial. As Fromm (2001) has put it, we must adapt to the world in which we find ourselves as a matter of self-preservation.

Our own roles within the groups of which we are part and, stemming from these, the identities which we take on for ourselves, are reflections of wider patterns of personal and social relationships within a set of institutional arrangements that impose a certain order on society. By participating within the world we reproduce the relationships and the ways of thinking about and looking at the world that are around us (Burr 1997). By engaging within the world, we give our assent to being part of that world. Through our daily lives, through the ways in which we feel, think and behave we put into practice and reinforce the social relations of the cultures to which we belong. By associating within family groups we put into practice and reinforce existing models of kinship; by buying from supermarkets we put into practice and reinforce existing models of production, distribution and consumption; by going to school or university we put into practice and reinforce existing models of education; by presenting ourselves as sets of symptoms requiring medical attention we put into practice and reinforce existing models of health care; by going to work we put into practice and reinforce existing models of labour, by rebelling and dropping out we put into practice and reinforce existing models of popular subculture (Fiske 1993).

There are certain ways of doing things that are imposed as constraints upon our development and certain ways of doing things that are considered right and wrong, appropriate and inappropriate, natural and unnatural, normal and abnormal. Very often these are presented to us as facts, beyond dispute; whereas they are really reflections of looking at the world in a particular way. What is presented to us as being natural, the right and proper way of doing things, of behaving according to the gender roles, the age roles, the ethnic roles, the disability roles ascribed to us, is not only not necessarily natural, but also not necessarily the best way of ordering and organizing life (Morris 1991). It reflects the particular type of culture that is held to be desirable by those who have power to shape and influence the world in which we live.

The ways in which we feel and think and behave toward ourselves and others are experienced as expressions of our individuality, but are, to a large extent, regulated by what is culturally acceptable within the social context in which we exist. This is why we expend a great deal of time and effort in presenting ourselves to the world around us as reliable normal, healthy, unlikely to cause trouble, motivated and with an attractive image (Fromm 1984). This is also, as Fromm points out, why individuals experience a profound fear of being perceived as different. We are free to express ourselves as individuals, certainly, but in order to experience ourselves as accepted, respected, integrated individuals whose skills and talents and abilities will be sought by potential employers, friends, partners and so on, we must accept that we are able to do this only within culturally acceptable boundaries. In order to fit in with the expectations of those around us, we must conform in our attitudes and behaviours. Drawing attention to ourselves is disapproved of and being perceived as 'not belonging' leads, all too frequently, to trouble.

Questions for discussion

1 In what ways do you think of yourself as different from others around you?
2 In what ways do you experience yourself as similar to those around you?
3 To what extent do you think that your perception of yourself is shaped by the way you think that others perceive you?

Models of disability

The medical model of disability provides a conceptual framework within which disability can be understood, assessed, experienced, planned for and justified. The central focus of this model lies in its location of disability as an individual problem tied to the functional limitations of the bodies of people with impairments. The medical model reflects wider cultural assumptions around individuality, personal autonomy and self-determination within a society in which great value is placed upon 'standing on your own two feet', 'staying one step ahead', 'standing up for yourself', 'walking tall' and 'making great strides' (Keith 1994: 57). The emphasis placed upon self-presentation as 'normal' arises out of a need to be perceived as being in control or disciplined. As the body is where nature and culture meet, and is the site where social relations and patterns of interactive behaviour are negotiated, it is the fore-most location for the struggle to gain and exercise control.

Physical impairment represents a threat to established notions of discipline and normality because it serves to draw attention to uncontrollable nature – to limitations placed upon the ability of humans to shape and organize the world around them as they wish. Impairment signifies disorder, indiscipline, unreli-ability (Davis 1995) and, as such, it is perceived as undesirable, something to be cured, overcome or hidden. Disabled people are under pressure to prove themselves; to demonstrate that the impact of their impairments is of minimal significance in making them who they are; to persuade others that they are doing their best to fit in, in spite of their unfortunate bodies (Stanton 1996).

The medical model is reinforced through wider cultural representation of disability and disabled people. Disabled commentators (Barnes 1994; Garland Thomson 1997) have drawn attention to the stereotypes – the poor, pathetic victim; the plucky, tragic but brave hero; and the evil, twisted villain with a chip on their shoulder – used widely within literature and film to depict dis-abled characters. The unquestioned assumption that disabled people have extra or 'special' needs for care, support and help is used to legitimize the separate provision of services in areas such as education, housing, public transport, training and employment. Within a medical model framework, the surrounding environment and culture within which impaired individuals are situated is regarded as unproblematic. The medical model reflects a frame-work of thinking about disability that has been and continues to be imposed by non-disabled people upon disabled people. It reflects and reinforces domi-nant ideas about individuals and their roles within society; it values con-formity and asserts the significance of self-reliance.

The Union of the Physically Impaired Against Segregation (UPIAS) devel-oped an alternative to the medical model which has become known as the social model of disability:

> Impairment: Lacking part or all of a limb, or having a defective limb, organ or mechanism of the body.

> Disability: The disadvantage or restriction of activity caused by a contem-porary social organisation which takes no or little account of people who have physical impairments and thus excludes them from participation in the mainstream of social activities.
>
> (UPIAS 1976: 14)

Impairment is, as in the medical model, identified as a physical characteristic but disability is reconstructed as a social and political process. Rather than being perceived as a problem arising from the limitations of people's with impairments, disability is recognized as being created by societies that are organized to suit the requirements of non-disabled people and which ignore the requirements of disabled people. Disability ceases to be something that a person *has*, and becomes instead something that is done to the person. To be disabled is to have experiences of being excluded and of being confronted on a daily basis by physical, environmental, legal, cultural and attitudinal barriers which limit opportunities for human experience. The definition by UPIAS (1976) was later extended by Disabled Peoples' International (DPI) to embrace intellectual impairments, sensory impairments and mental distress (Barnes 1994). It is further extended by Thomas to take into account psycho-emotional well-being:

> Disability is a form of social oppression involving the social imposition of restrictions of activity on people with impairments and the socially engendered undermining of their psycho-emotional well-being.
>
> (Thomas 1999: 60)

Oliver (1990) draws attention to the emergence of disability as a result of processes of industrialization in the nineteenth century. In pre-industrial, feudal society most work had been organized around agriculture or small-scale industry where people with impairments had often been able to contribute. New factory-based production forces, however, led to the emergence of detailed attention to speed, discipline, timekeeping and production norms. As surveillance focused increasingly upon the monitoring of behaviours of individuals within work processes, there emerged the construction of 'the able-bodied worker'. Against this norm, it became possible to identify and remove individuals who did not match up to the requirements of modern production processes. Labelled as unfit, sick or incapable, people with impairments found themselves increasingly segregated from mainstream society and confined within workhouses, asylums, hospitals, colonies and special schools.

Most of the towns and cities in which we live today are those which grew and developed during the industrial revolution. Provision for the requirements of the communities who lived within them (transport systems, education systems, places of work, housing provision, places of leisure, entertainment and worship) was similarly based on the premise that people with impairments would have their needs met elsewhere. There was little point seen in taking their needs into account in the design and delivery of mainstream social provision.

The central point of the social model of disability is that it provides a critique from which disabled people can argue that the social exclusion they have experienced has gone on for far too long. Disabled people want the same chances and opportunities in life as non-disabled people: to gain an education, employment, to live in affordable accessible housing, to have relationships, to be able to make their own decisions about the issues that affect their lives. The importance of the social model of disability is that, as a model providing an alternative understanding of the experience and reality of disability, it has given disabled people a basis on which to organize themselves collectively. Using the social model as a basis for explanation, disabled people have been drawing attention to the real problems of disability: the barriers they face; the patronizing attitudes they have to deal with; the low expectations that are invested in them; and the limited options available to them. The social model has also been the foundation for demands to be included in society.

While the social model has proved an invaluable tool, there have been some disabled writers who suggest that the disabled people's movement has overemphasized the discrimination inherent in disabling relationships at the expense of acknowledging the significance of impairment within people's lives (Crow 1996; Shakespeare 1996). For example, Thomas states:

> For some, the social model focuses too heavily, or exclusively, on socio-structural barriers (determining access to life's material necessities) and downplays or ignores the cultural and experiential dimensions of disablism.
>
> (Thomas 1999: 24)

Crow (1996) acknowledges the reasons underlying this emphasis, stating that too much focus on impairment may place disabled people in danger of being perceived as weakening their own case and acknowledging the validity of medical approaches to disability. She has suggested, however, that there needs to be more open discussion about the nature of impairment. A renewed social model of disability, she argues, would allow for a more complete understanding of disability and impairment as social constructs and would recognize an individual's experiences of their body over time and in different circumstances.

Crow (1996) calls for 'a new norm' which carries an expectation that there will be a wide range of attributes within a population, and an acceptance and valuing of difference. A greater acceptance of the diversity that exists among individuals and more appropriate provision for the inclusion of diversity within the mainstream will, she suggests, lead to a lessening of the need to place labels of impairment upon individuals. She emphasizes the need to bring discussion about impairment into greater prominence in order that the social change that disabled people aim to bring about is genuinely inclusive.

Questions for discussion

1 What impact do you think the medical model has on the way that non-disabled people regard disabled people?
2 What impact do you think the medical model has on the way disabled people regard themselves?
3 Why do you think disabled people have rejected the medical model?

Dyslexia: disability or difference?

The word 'dyslexia' derives from the Greek language and literally means 'difficulty with words'. In the first half of the twentieth century it was referred to as 'word blindness'. It is now recognized, however, that many people labelled dyslexic have difficulty dealing with numbers and understanding other symbols such as musical notation (British Dyslexia Association 2002). People may also experience problems with short-term memory and in organizing their work and their time.

Dyslexia has been described as a genetic difference in brain structure and function which gives rise to specific learning difficulties (Dyslexia Institute 2002). About 10 per cent of the population have some degree of dyslexia varying from severe to mild and with huge variations, from person to person, in the problems encountered. It is more common in males than females.

Many individuals labelled as dyslexic have been shown to be advantaged in terms of visual and perceptual skills and in their ability to think creatively and laterally (British Dyslexia Association 2002). They tend to thrive in occupations such as architecture, engineering, art and graphic design. For this reason dyslexia is often referred to as a 'difference' rather than a deficit, impairment or disability.

For this case study we interviewed Jack Osborn. Jack was born in 1943 but was not labelled as dyslexic until 1996 when he enrolled on an undergraduate degree. The underlying explanatory model that was used to describe Jack's difficulties as a child was in terms of his intellect. Like many people with dyslexia Jack was described as 'thick' and 'slow'. He said:

> I can distinctly remember Dad sitting there teaching me the times tables by rote, and learning how to spell sort of parrot fashion, and that's the only way that it went in . . . You were put into the slow stream, right at the bottom, and you were expected to leave at 16 and that was it. I did science, woodwork and metalwork. The school that I went to told me that there was no way I would ever get a GCE [General Certificate of Education].

These experiences did not, however, dent Jack's self-esteem. He said:

> I didn't think anything of it. You left school at the age of 16, you got a job, you did your job and that was it. I think at that age you're more interested in drinking and girls and it didn't hold me back with any of that.

Jack's main difficulty concerns the manipulation of numbers but he had no way of explaining this to himself, or to others, until he was assessed as being dyslexic at the age of 53. He explained how this happened and the effect it had on him:

> It was first discovered when I was doing a foundation course up at the university. The maths tutor there said 'I can't work you out, I don't think you're thick, I think you might be dyslexic' and I said 'What's dyslexic?' Anyway, she got me assessed and the report came back saying 'Yes, dyslexic'. To me that explained an awful lot. I was walking around in shock for weeks. It explained why I couldn't do the maths on this course. On everything else I was getting As and Bs.

Jack does not view dyslexia as a deficit or an impairment but rather as part of human diversity:

I look at it that everyone is different. Dyslexia, like autism, is something that is different from the norm and because of this we do need treating slightly differently. We're not the same as other people, we never will be. We look at life in a different way. Therefore we can offer society different things, different approaches, different values to that of the norm – we're supposed to be artists, we're supposed to see things laterally. As soon as I have to deal with three-dimensional objects I'm good at that whereas other people may run into a block. I was always good at the practical.

He also sees the label 'dyslexia' as being part of a wider tendency to label 'difference':

There's so many things these days that are recognised but they're only facets of human psychology really. I mean 'what is normal?' Do I want to be normal? No, I don't want to be part of the grey, amorphous mass. I'm me. I'm an individual. But we're never happy with ourselves are we? We always wish we were something different, something better – taller, wavy haired, blond or whatever. But it's nice to know what dyslexia is. I wish they'd told me earlier, but they hadn't invented it then.

Jack feels that the main effect dyslexia has had on his life were his inability to gain promotion. He said:

It's affected my life because I would have liked promotion. I'm sure it prevented my promotion to a higher technical officer. The annual report always said 'not a very good communicator, the written reports could be better'.

When he retired Jack decided to study and began by taking GCSE (General Certificate of Secondary Education) courses in English and maths. His earlier experiences of the educational system did not deter him:

I remember thinking 'oh dear, I'm having the same problems as I had last time', but it was more of a social occasion than a learning occasion. We were all adults. It was a pleasure to go. It got me out of the house.

This led on to the successful completion of a BSc degree in Maritime Environmental Management, although there were initial problems:

I started off doing a bachelor of engineering degree up at the university and I was discovered dyslexic on the foundation year. I thought 'I'm not going to survive this' so I transferred here. I started off here with Maritime Studies but I was obliquely advised that it may not be the thing for me so I looked at what else was on offer and thought 'if I do that I've got no sums at all'. I don't feel disadvantaged on the course that I'm doing but with some subjects I would be severely disadvantaged. I find it a thundering nuisance. I thoroughly enjoy maths yet because of the dyslexia I can't do the number shuffling as well as I would want to.

Now that the difficulties Jack experiences can be explained and have been labelled he is given help which he never received in the past:

> In exams I'm given extra time and I've also been given a computer because nobody can read my writing. I have a sticker that I can put on the work so that tutors are aware that I'm dyslexic. They really couldn't be more helpful.

Despite the predictions of his teachers when Jack was a child, he is now studying a Master of Science degree in International Maritime Studies.

Questions for discussion

1 What explanatory models of dyslexia are identified in this account? How would dyslexia be viewed from a medical model? How would dyslexia be viewed from a social model?
2 What would be the resulting policies and practices founded on these explanatory models?
3 Do you think dyslexia is a disability or simply a difference? On what basis do you make this judgement?

Debate activity

Debate the proposition: The medical model has played a significant role in the creation of disability. The following quotations may provide you with a starting point.

> Disability is defined in this section and throughout the book as: . . . a loss or deviation, in either a qualitative or quantitative way, of the ability to perform an activity or behaviour, taking into account age, gender, and environment . . . Disabilities happen to a whole person, not to a particular body part, organ, system or cell. They are characterised by the activity that is affected, rather than by the nature of the health problem causing them. Thus disabilities are often described using verbs, for example, a walking disability, a seeing disability, an information-processing disability.
>
> (McColl and Bickenbach 1998: 55–6)

Disabled Apartheid

The municipal might of Victorian Architecture – No need for a sign saying

CRIPPLES KEEP OUT

When triumphal stone flights of stairs
Smugly bar the way to
the art gallery
the library
the committee meeting.

Not that it was deliberate you understand,
They were far too nice for that,
They simply forgot
To think that we might want to
Get in

Take our share
Play our part
Claim some space.
Perhaps they had in mind
That our place
Was outside
With begging bowl in hand.

(Napolitano 1992)

Further reading

Barnes, C. and Mercer, G. (eds) (1996) *Exploring the Divide: Illness and Disability.* Leeds: The Disability Press.

Barnes, C., Mercer, M. and Shakespeare, T. (1999) *Exploring Disability: A Sociological Introduction.* Cambridge: Polity Press.

Burr, V. (1997) *An Introduction to Social Constructionism.* London: Routledge.

Fiske, J. (1993) *Power Plays, Power Works.* London: Verso.

3

What is 'disability studies'?

What is knowledge?

This chapter concerns the nature and development of disability studies as an academic discipline. The first section of the chapter broadly examines the nature of knowledge and focuses in particular on the development of women's studies. The second section of the chapter explores the rise of disability studies and examines the many controversies that ensue in developing and maintaining it as an academic discipline in universities. In the third section of the chapter a case study of a disability studies programme is described. The case study includes a small survey of the opinions of second year students who are following the programme.

People in every culture have bodies of knowledge by which they organize their thoughts, behaviour and lives, but there is little agreement among different groups about what is 'right' or 'wrong', 'true' or 'false'. In western society, for example, the birth of twins is regarded as a biological phenomenon with no moral overtones, but for the Punan Bah of Central Borneo it is a social disgrace and a sign of an insatiable sexual urge (Nicolaisen 1995). Knowledge is thus culturally relative and changes over time.

Explanatory and moral frameworks also change over time within the same society. In western society, for example, we are influenced more by scientific ideas, and less by religious ideas, than we were in the past. Glover and Strawbridge (1985) illustrate this point with a medical example:

if a doctor in our society started to practise exorcism in a attempt to cast out demons from patients, we should count this unreasonable. It is likely that we would seek causes for the doctor's behaviour in terms of his or her mental health. However, when the belief in demons as a cause of ill-health was widespread in our society, it would have been perfectly reasonable to attempt to cast them out.

(Glover and Strawbridge 1985: 63)

Even the most 'objective' knowledge from the past can look quaint when viewed from the perspective of our particular culture and place in history, for events can be fully understood only when they are situated within a social, cultural, political and historical context. As Marx and Engels (1968: 181) state, 'it is not the consciousness of men that determine their existence, but, on the contrary, their social existence that determines their consciousness.' According to Potter (2000), for example, colonial rule was, at least in part, established and maintained by a powerful set of beliefs which were accepted and endorsed by those who were oppressed.

There is an old maxim that 'knowledge is power'. The relationship between knowledge and power is central to many sociological theories. Weber, for example, linked political power to class advantage which he believed was maintained by structures of kinship and education (Fulcher and Scott 1999). Foucault spoke in terms of 'discourses' to explain how ideas and knowledge are produced, reproduced and sustained through talk and writing (Clarke and Cochrane 1998). Feminists, on the other hand, have argued that even such seemingly personal feelings as romantic love can be understood in term of power inequalities between the sexes (Langford 1996).

Power has the potential to be manifested in policy, practice and behaviour which, in turn, helps to construct and sustain what is felt to be 'true'. Professionals may, for example, mystify knowledge in order to maintain their privileged position (Hugman 1991) and people, particularly women in poorer countries, are kept powerless by policies and practices which maintain their illiteracy (Parker and Wilson 2000). Governments have the power to devise school curricula where they emphasize particular subjects and values. In the Education Act 1870, for example, needlework was a compulsory subject for girls in England and Wales (McCoy 1998) and the present National Curriculum for schools in England and Wales, which was introduced in the Education Act 1988, is very conventional. It does not, for example, include subjects such as politics, economics and sociology.

If more than one set of beliefs about a particular phenomenon exist within a society, the explanatory model of the most powerful group will be validated as 'true' and superior to the explanatory models of others. As Marx (1955: 47) states, 'the ideas of the ruling class are in every epoch the ruling ideas.' In societies where people have access to varying perspectives, and sufficient power to promote their point of view, there is likely to be conflict among different bodies of knowledge and the possibility of a 'paradigm shift' as one set of beliefs becomes more influential than another. As Lewis (2002: 35) comments, 'While one voice or meaning occupies a position of dominance there are always other meanings struggling to assume ascendancy.'

New systems of belief can seriously challenge the existing order. Copernicus (1473–1543), for instance, insisted that the earth revolved around the sun, rather than the sun around the earth, yet despite a sound theory he found little support among other astronomers in his lifetime. Similarly Darwin (1809–82) enraged the religious establishment with his theory of natural selection which opposed the ideology of divine creation.

In the 1970s feminism became a powerful ideology which challenged most frameworks of knowledge because of the exclusion of women in its production. Fulcher and Scott (1999) state:

> The main thrust of feminist thought has been the claim that knowledge is related to divisions of sex and gender. Put simply men and women have different experiences and so have different standpoints from which they construct their knowledge . . . Feminists, then, suggest that mainstream theory must be seen as malestream theory. It is rooted in patriarchal relations that embody male power over women and that establish the male standpoint on knowledge.
>
> (Fulcher and Scott 1999: 63)

Since the late 1960s women's studies has become established as an academic discipline in higher education and is offered at both undergraduate and post-graduate level in many universities. It has also become a distinct strand within studies of the majority world after many years of marginalization (Pearson 2000). The first degree courses in women's studies developed in the late 1960s in the USA and became a substantial presence during the 1970s and 1980s in many countries including Britain. Easton (1996) explains that:

> Women's studies . . . involves the way gender relations have operated in social life in the past and the present. It encompasses the study of representation of women's experiences in, for example, literature, language and religion. It includes the study of concepts used to differentiate women and men, such as femininity and masculinity. In addition it examines theoretical perspectives on all the above, particularly those drawn from feminist theory.
>
> (Easton 1996: 5)

Women's studies has radically revised many academic fields. It is interdisciplinary, overtly political and recognizes the value of personal experience. It has been at the forefront of the development of feminist theory and new research approaches. The rise of the feminist movement has thus created new knowledge and insights. The same can be said of other social movements such as Gay Pride and the Green movement. This is not to imply that issues of power are absent. Women's studies, for example, may not welcome the input of men and it can be argued that the ideas purported in new social movements are initially shaped by a powerful, well-educated, social elite. Working-class and Black feminists, for example, have criticized feminism for ignoring their cultural differences and some believe that they may have more in common with working-class and Black men than with white feminists (Smith 1996).

Although women's studies has expanded over the years in terms of courses, tutors, students and textbooks, Griffin (1998) is cautious about its future. Women's studies, as an academic subject, is still relatively marginalized. There are, for example, very few women's studies departments, with most courses being based within other academic disciplines. The number of posts specific to women's studies is few, with even fewer senior posts, which leads to poor career prospects and a fear of being marginalized. There is frequently lack of institutional support and funding for research and the multidisciplinary nature of women's studies does not fit well with traditional university structures, which tend to be subject specific. Over recent years student numbers have been static or falling which, as well as the above factors, may be due to competition from 'gender studies' and a dissemination of the ideas emanating from women's studies into other academic disciplines. Despite this Wise (1996) believes that women's studies is a major vehicle for the dissemination of feminist ideas and an important form of feminist activism.

Questions for discussion

1 Give some examples from your own life that involved knowledge as power, both when you had power over others and when others had power over you.
2 What do these experiences tell you about the relationship between knowledge and power?
3 If all knowledge is embedded within a social, historical, political and cultural context, can anything be said to be 'true'?

The emergence of disability studies

Disability studies is a relatively new area of academic inquiry (Gleeson 1997) which is interdisciplinary and diverse, drawing on sociology, linguistics, economics, anthropology, politics, history, psychology and media studies (Pfeiffer and Yoshida 1995). Disability studies has been promoted largely by disabled activists and disabled academics from various disciplines, particularly sociology. Their work has had much to offer disability studies in the development of theory (Barnes et al. 1999; Thomas 1999); the analysis of professional ideologies and practices (Davis 1993; Priestley 1999); the examination of the disabled people's movement (Driedger 1989; Campbell and Oliver 1996); disability equality training (Swain and Lawrence 1994); and the development of new approaches to research (Rioux and Bach 1994; Barnes and Mercer 1997). There are now several master's degree courses in disability studies in Britain and a growing academic literature, including the international journal *Disability and Society*, which was launched in 1986. Finkelstein (1998: 33) defines disability studies as 'the study of disabled people's lifestyles and aspirations' and Pfeiffer and Yoshida (1995) state that disability studies

> reframes the study of disability by focusing on it as a social phenomenon, social construct, metaphor and culture utilising a minority group model . . . This focus shifts the emphasis away from a prevention/treatment/remediation paradigm to a social/cultural/political paradigm.
>
> (Pfeiffer and Yoshida 1995: 480)

Although disability studies encompasses many sociological perspectives, for example Marxism and feminism, in its quest to explain disability, a rejection of any explanatory model that locates disability within the person is a common and central feature (Paterson and Hughes 2000; Albrecht et al. 2001).

Before the advent of disability studies much of the theoretical analysis of disability took place within medicine and psychology where the voices of disabled people themselves were rarely heard (Oliver 1996a). In this context disability is viewed in terms of biology and psychological processes and mechanisms. It is regarded as an individual tragedy rather than a social phenomenon (Oliver 1996b; Gleeson 1997). This view of disability is still dominant in most societies and has inhibited alternative meanings (Linton 1998a). Omansky Gordon and Rosenblum (2001) emphasize the links between disability studies and the study of race, gender and sexual orientation.

The academic discipline of sociology has come under criticism from disabled people for ignoring disability as a social phenomenon. Barton (1996: 3), for example, contends that although 'the sociological task is to make connections between, for example, structural conditions and the lived reality of people in particular settings', mainstream sociology has paid scant attention to disabled people. Sociologists have viewed disability in medical and psychological terms and have thus perceived it as non-sociological. They have ignored the disabled people's movement as a legitimate area of study and the work of disabled sociologists is rarely mentioned in mainstream sociological texts (Barton 1996; Barnes 1998). Finkelstein (1998) believes that:

> Disability studies . . . clearly could not emerge within the bounds of any discipline that had percolated out of 'normal' academic studies, simply because we had been removed from this arena . . . What was needed to open the door to the radically new approach of 'disability studies' was the infusion of ideas directly from the experiences of disabled people.
>
> (Finkelstein 1998: 32, 35)

Disability studies has yet to gain the status of, for example, women's studies because of its recent origins and the neglect of disability within sociology and every other academic discipline including history, art and science (Linton 1998a). This can make funding for research and teaching initiatives difficult and the disabling physical and social environment of universities can pose great difficulties for disabled academics (of whom there are few) and disabled students alike.

Pfeiffer and Yoshida (1995) believe that people working within the framework of disability studies are often considered to be 'outsiders' in academic life but that disability studies is an exciting new field of academic inquiry which is at the frontier of knowledge and which will make a difference to society beyond disability. Linton (1998a) asserts that:

> A disability studies perspective adds a critical dimension to thinking about issues such as autonomy, competence, wholeness, independence/

dependence, health, physical appearance, aesthetics, community and notions of progress and perfection – issues that pervade every aspect of the civic and pedagogic culture.

(Linton 1998a: 118)

Despite the many positive issues that can be raised regarding the nature and growth of disability studies, a number of controversies have been voiced. Central to these is the issue of who controls and who should control disability studies. Is it controlled by representative groups of disabled people? Is it controlled by a powerful, well-educated elite of disabled people who have academic posts in universities? Or is it controlled by funders and those who have power over university budgets and curricula? This controversy was voiced by Oliver (1999) towards the end of his career as a researcher and academic:

> I am the main beneficiary of this work . . . my own work leaves me confronted with a certain amount of existential guilt which I cannot ignore or wish away . . . When we set up research programmes, persuade our organizations to take a specific interest in disability issues and bid into funded initiatives . . . we are instrumental in the production of a particular set of social relations . . . I can no longer pretend that adopting any of the above strategies is the best we can do in current circumstances or that it is better than doing nothing. Because of the oppressive structures in which we are located, such actions inevitably keep that oppression in place.
>
> (Oliver 1999: 185, 187–8)

Academics in disability studies can, and do, involve representative groups of disabled people in the planning and delivery of courses, but university rules (regarding assessment for example) mean that representative groups are less powerful than the disabled academics themselves. It can also be argued that disability studies, and the disabled people's movement generally, is dominated by a white, male elite (Morris 1991; Hill 1994).

Another controversy concerns where disability studies should be located within the university structure of faculties and departments. Disability studies often sits, rather uncomfortably, in departments of 'health studies', 'social care' and 'rehabilitation' where health care academics, with a medical orientation to disability, may be eager to get involved. Departments of 'social sciences' may appear to be more appropriate and yet, as we have seen, sociology pays scant attention to disability while psychology takes an individualistic stance.

A further dilemma is whether non-disabled people should teach disability studies. Similar arguments can, of course, be raised about men teaching women's studies and white people conducting race equality training. Other anxieties concern the ways in which ideas emanating from disability studies may be used (by health professionals for example) and whether, in the face of small numbers of students enrolling on disability studies courses, it would be more pragmatic to 'disseminate' the ideas throughout other university programmes. This may also provide interesting opportunities to engage in dialogue with other disciplines, such as history and cultural studies, which are relevant to disability studies. Linton, however, is suspicious of this approach. She states: 'The health and occupational therapy programs' appropriation of disability studies compromises the integrity of a field designed to explicate disability as a social, political and cultural phenomenon' (Linton 1998a: 133).

It can also be argued that if disability studies is marginalized within other subjects areas there is the danger that complex ideas will be misunderstood or inadequately explored leading to more, rather than less, prejudice. Finkelstein (1998) cites the rise of 'community care', as an academic discipline, as a 'pernicious influence' on the growth of disability studies.

A further controversy in disability studies is the extent to which impairment and personal experience of disability should be included. Paterson and Hughes (2000: 35) contend that the 'dualistic view of the social and the biological as binary opposites is one of the maxims on which disability studies is founded' and that the embodied experience of disability has been denied. The social model of disability is, however, constantly developing and various theorists, for example Morris (1991) and Crow (1996), have attempted to incorporate the sociology of impairment into the social model of disability and to consider the individual experiences of disabled people in order to develop a broader account.

A broader understanding would also be gained by paying more attention to the experiences and writings of disabled people in the majority world. As Priestley (2001) states:

> the academic literature of disability studies consistently privileges minority world accounts (especially those from Western Europe and North America) . . . Majority world perspectives do exist . . . However such contributions are rarely cited within the academic literature of disability studies.
>
> (Priestley 2001: 3, 4)

There may, for example, be struggles for, rather than against, special education, rehabilitation and sheltered workshops in many majority world countries where the alternative is no education, health care or employment and no welfare state. There are, however, numerous commonalties among disabled people throughout the world (Priestley 2001).

Questions for discussion

1 Who should be in control of disability studies?
2 What similarities and differences are there between disability studies and women's studies in terms of scope, development and struggle?
3 Should disability studies be an academic subject in its own right or should it be integrated into other disciplines?

Disability studies in practice

The first disability studies course at the University of Northumbria had its initial intake in 1993. This was a postgraduate certificate course from which students could progress to a master's degree although this was not specific to disability studies. A multidisciplinary team of university tutors from across the Faculty of Health, Social Work and Education planned the programme of study. They included two tutors from each of the following areas: education, social work, nursing, occupational therapy and the Disability Research Unit. At that time two members of the teaching team identified themselves as disabled. Two others later became impaired and regarded themselves as disabled people as well.

The postgraduate certificate course took place one evening per week over one academic year. It operated for three years. Approximately 26 students took the course, of whom about 5 were disabled. Most students were professionals working with disabled people in various capacities. A small number of students were neither disabled nor professionals. These included two sales assistants who worked in large department stores.

The course that is the subject of this case study developed from this postgraduate certificate course which was discontinued due to a low level of recruitment. The official number for a viable course was over 15 each year and this course did not attract the requisite number of students. A small survey was undertaken to find out why it had not recruited well and the biggest problem seemed to be the course fees.

The new course, which at the time of writing has its fourth intake of students, is a part route to a BA joint honours degree programme. Half of the programme comprises disability studies and students can select the other half from several subject areas including 'childhood studies' and 'professional practice studies'. Consultations were made with disabled people including a disabled academic, a disabled access officer and a representative of a local organization of disabled people. Two disabled people produced the final version of the course.

Approximately 20 students have studied the course each year. About a quarter were mature students (over 21), 4 were disabled, and almost all were female. Some students had disabled family members and most had experience of working with disabled people.

Below are selected extracts from the course documentation that is available to all students and staff.

Philosophy of the Part Route
The part route in disability studies explores the experiences and lives of disabled people. Students will examine the attitudinal, environmental and structural barriers that disabled people face in a non-disabled social world. We would stress that this is *not* a programme about medical conditions.

Disability studies owes its existence to the development of the disabled people's movement and the social model of disability developed within the movement. Because the part route has been developed in response to these broader social and political movements, it is deemed essential that disabled people have majority roles in the planning, delivery and continuous evolution of the course.

The philosophy of the part route is founded on the belief that the social model of disability is an academic discipline in its own right. This academic discipline is relatively new, as with Peace Studies, Gender Studies and Gay Studies. Both students and academic staff will see themselves as participants in an exciting and challenging developing field of study.

The Aim of the Disability Studies Part Route
The part route is rooted within, and shall reflect, the development of the disabled people's movement and the social model of disability developed within the movement.

Therefore within this context the objectives are that the part route will:

1 Enable critical thought, reflection and personal growth.
2 Explore the experiences and lives of disabled people by examining the barriers that disabled people face in the social world.
3 Take the social model as the foundation for an enquiry based approach to the study of disability in a social world.

The structure of the course is as follows:

Year One
Disability Equality Training, Study Skills, Personal and Social Perspectives (double unit), Historical Perspectives on Disability, Perspectives of Disabled People.

Year Two
Disability and Lifestyle, Families and Relationships, Barriers, Rights, Politics and Policy (double unit), Disability Research, Impairment in a Social World (optional unit).

Year Three
Professional Perspectives (optional unit), Investigating Services, Barriers and Rights (double unit), Critical Issues and Current Debates in Disability Studies, Dissertation (double unit).

At the time of writing, the course is taught by one full-time professor and two part-time lecturers, two of whom are disabled. There is also substantial input from two non-disabled lecturers, one with a background in occupational therapy and the other in radiotherapy. The course team invite visiting lecturers, including representatives of local organizations of disabled people, to take part.

As part of this case study a questionnaire was distributed to students who were in the second year of the programme at the time of writing. Fifteen students completed the questionnaire. Although there were some criticisms, all took an essentially positive stance towards the course. Two of the group considered themselves to be disabled, though neither had an impairment. All were female. One, who identified herself as 'disabled', wrote 'Everyone is disabled by society. Always needing someone to rely on.'

The first question asked:

> What is 'Disability Studies'? Please give your definition in a few sentences or phrases.

The following is a typical answer:

> A course aimed at giving an understanding of the social model of disability. Understanding that disability is with society's attitudes not the person, therefore moving the focus from the individual to the environment and society.

Another of the questions asked,

> In what ways has your understanding of what Disability Studies is changed since you started the course?

The majority of students referred to the social model in contrast to the medical model. One student wrote:

> To challenge professionals whereas prior to my studies professional viewpoints seemed to be the be all and end all.

Another wrote:

> It is completely different to my expectations, and my views and opinions towards disability have changed, broadened and moved away from the medical approach.

A third suggested:

> I no longer look at a person with an impairment and feel pity.

In response to the question, 'What are you hoping to do when you graduate?', most students cited working with disabled children in a professional role. One wrote:

> Not sure yet. Hopefully something along the lines of social work with children within the autistic spectrum, or people who are labelled with the term schizophrenia.

The students were also asked:

> What do you think about the involvement of non-disabled people (as either students or tutors) in Disability Studies?

All asserted the importance of the involvement of both disabled and non-disabled people. One wrote:

Important to have both disabled and non-disabled – there is still isolation and segregation – gives good insight to non-disabled people just how much attitudes and environment form barriers. It's important that non-disabled work alongside disabled people on disability studies.

This joint honours degree is one of the few courses in the faculty which is not a 'professional education' course. The faculty offers professional education courses for teachers, social workers, nurses, occupational therapists, physiotherapists and midwives. There is now a recognized group of disability studies tutors who provide input to other courses, particularly in occupational therapy and physiotherapy.

Questions for discussion

1 What is 'disability studies'? Give your definition in a few sentences or phrases.
2 What do you think about the involvement of non-disabled people (as either students or tutors) in disability studies?
3 In what ways might a disability studies course, as described above, further disabled people's struggles for change and in what ways might the course inhibit or 'colonize' the field of disability through the domination of non-disabled people.

Debate activity

Debate the proposition: Disability studies is a clearly defined academic discipline which has emerged from the views and experiences of disabled people. The following quotations may provide you with a starting point:

> there is a tendency within the social model of disability to deny the experience of our own bodies, insisting that our physical differences and restrictions are entirely socially created. While environmental barriers and social attitudes are a crucial part of our experience of disability – and do indeed disable us – to suggest that this is all there is to it is to deny the very personal experience of physical or intellectual restrictions, of illness, of the fear of dying.
>
> (Morris 1991: 10)

> If a person's physical pain is the reason they are unhappy then there is nothing the disability movement can do about it. All that BCODP (British Council of Disabled People) can do is facilitate the politicisation of disabled people around these issues.
>
> (Vasey 1992a: 43)

Further reading

Albrecht, G.L., Seelman, K.D. and Bury, M. (2001) Introduction: the formation of disability studies, in G.L. Albrecht, K.D. Seelman and M. Bury (eds) *Handbook of Disability Studies*. London: Sage.

Finkelstein, V. (1998) Emancipating disability studies, in T. Shakespeare (ed.) *The Disability Reader: Social Science Perspectives*. London: Cassell.

Linton, S. (1998) Disability studies/not disability studies, *Disability and Society*, 13(4): 525–40.

Oliver, M. (1996) A sociology of disability or a disablist sociology?, in L. Barton (ed.) *Disability and Society: Emerging Issues and Insights*. London: Longman.

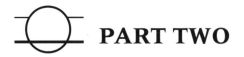 **PART TWO**

VALUES AND IDEOLOGIES

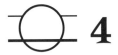 **4**

Controlling life?

Colin Goble

The genetic revolution

In this chapter I shall focus on developments in genetic medicine and their implications for disabled people. First, I shall look at some of the broad social issues relating to the so-called 'genetic revolution'. The basics of the science itself will then be outlined as a basis for understanding its medical applications. The 'curative' and 'preventive' approaches to genetic medicine will then be outlined. Brief reference to the history of scientific techniques applied to heredity and disability will be made in order to place issues and concerns about its current usage in context. Current concerns about the use of, and social meaning attached to prenatal screening for genetic 'abnormality' will then be explored. Finally I shall look at a case study of 'Joanne' and her knowledge of the situation of people with Huntington's disease in order to gain some insight into the experience of living with genetic disease in our society.

We are currently living in an era of biotechnological revolution rivalling that of information technology in its potential economic and cultural impact. In areas like agriculture and medicine extravagant claims are being made for genetic technologies with the alleged potential to save humanity from starvation and evolutionary meltdown. We are, we are told, on the verge of taking control from nature of our own evolutionary destiny (Silver 1998).

For many people however, far from invoking utopian daydreams, such claims raise deep fears about the use and control of such technologies, particularly in the hands of transnational corporations working to aggressive, profit-oriented agendas in a deregulated, globalized economy (Ho 1999). Certainly, there is an eerie sense that we have heard similar claims before from scientists and politicians eager to associate themselves with cutting-edge technology. It is not so long ago that claims of universal social and economic benefit were being made for nuclear technology. Now, in the post Three Mile

Island, Chernobyl and Sellafield era, such claims look almost fanciful, and the reputation of the science that made them is tarnished. A new public scepticism is apparent. Across Europe we have recently seen a consumer reaction against genetically modified food which has made the UK and some other countries an effective no-go zone (at present) for the companies producing it. A key part in this consumer reaction has been a lack of trust in the evidence produced to back the technology, and a deep-seated unease that commercially driven science is messing with things that are fundamental to our biological and ecological well-being.

One area where there appears to be less concern however, is in the medical application of genetic technology. Medicine, despite recent public image troubles, is still held in esteem surpassing that of other sectors of applied science in our society. This is enhanced when medical science makes claims that include the potential eradication of genetic disease. I shall go on to examine such claims later, but first it may be helpful to give a brief outline of some of the basic principles of genetics in order to inform subsequent discussion.

Genes are most easily understood as the biochemical instructions governing the development and functioning of cells. As a British Medical Association (1998) publication puts it,

> genes provide the instructions for our development from a fertilised egg (oocyte) to a fully grown adult and continue, throughout our lives, to provide the information necessary for everyday maintenance and functioning of our bodies. Genes are sections of DNA (deoxyribonucleic acid) which are contained in the chromosomes passed on from our parents at conception.
>
> (British Medical Association 1998: 28)

Genes have been likened to the information imprinted on cassette tape when a recording is made. Apart from sperm or egg (so-called 'germ') cells that contain 23 chromosomes, human cells contain 46 chromosomes, 23 inherited from each parent. Except in the case of identical twins, everyone inherits a unique mix of genetic material from their parents. The biological sex of an individual is decided by their inheritance of X and Y chromosomes from their parents. Mothers always contribute an X chromosome, but fathers can contribute either an X (for a girl) or a Y (for a boy).

The biochemical processes involved in genetic inheritance are complex, and errors in transmission are not infrequent. Often these errors, described in biological jargon as 'mutations', have little or no visible impact, and their accumulated effects are, in fact, a vital part of the mechanism by which species evolve. However some mutations produce dramatic effects. These range from the immediately fatal, resulting usually in miscarriage, to those that produce 'atypical' physiological development. These effects also range widely, from the relatively minor and invisible, like colour blindness, to the highly visible, like extremes in physical stature, to those which are threatening to survival, such as cystic fibrosis. The degree of impairment experienced as a result is also highly variable, with individuals with similar genetic profiles, such as an extra twenty-first chromosome in people with Down's syndrome, varying tremendously in both physiological and cognitive capacities.

In western societies these 'atypicalities' have often been pathologized and result in negatively valued characteristics, such as intellectual, physical or sensory impairment. The promise of genetic medicine is that it will give us the ability to 'select' those characteristics we value, and 'select out' those characteristics we do not. It is this emphasis on selection of characteristics on which the project of genetic science in medicine is primarily based. This is being pursued in two ways. The first is 'gene therapies', that is the attempt to manipulate genetic material in order to control the expression of characteristics. This approach attempts to prevent negative, or disease generating, characteristics and to enhance positive, or health-promoting, ones. This can be called the 'curative' approach. The second approach involves identifying genetic 'markers' related to disorders so that women at risk of carrying a genetically 'abnormal' infant can be identified and screened. The claim made here is that women/parents can then make the choice about whether to continue with the pregnancy, or whether to terminate it. This is the 'preventive' approach.

There is widespread consensus that these goals of medicine are good in that they will work to the benefit of individuals and society by ensuring that more people have 'desirable', and fewer people 'undesirable' characteristics. At work here is an implicit acceptance of Darwinian evolutionary theory with its central tenet of 'natural selection'. This holds that species evolve to 'fit' their environment as individuals displaying adaptive characteristics tend to survive and breed more successfully than those that do not. Some have argued that the success of human beings in conquering infectious disease has meant that this selective pressure is no longer able to function. The claim is, that for humanity to retain its 'fitness' as a species, we need to take on this selective role ourselves, and that genetic technology will facilitate this process (Silver 1998). This raises many questions about the extent to which children will be 'designed' to fit dominant social and cultural conceptions of desirability, and also about who will be able to access such technology. Other issues have been raised about the control and privacy of genetic information. These concerns tend to be countered by geneticists and the biotechnology industry, however, by reference to potential benefits, including the eradication of impairment. It is to such claims that we will now turn.

Questions for discussion

1 Why are some people concerned about the development of biotechnology for commercial gain?
2 How might some sections of society use Darwinian evolutionary theory to explain their own social position?
3 Why are some genetically related characteristics regarded as desirable whilst others are regarded as forms of disease?

Genetic medicine and disability

Medical attempts to eradicate disability are not new. The historic rise of scientific knowledge lent new power to ancient prejudices by creating rational arguments, based on statistical evidence, to underpin social policy and practice towards disabled people (Davis 1997). Eugenics emerged in nineteenth-century Britain based on Darwinian theory which fitted well with the self-perceptions of social elites who saw in it both a justification of their own social and political status, and a rationale for the control of groups whom they perceived to be a threat. Social Darwinists coined the phrase 'survival of the fittest' and helped develop influential policies that resulted in the segregation and sterilization of many disabled people (Ryan and Thomas 1987; Russell 1998). The most notorious programme was that pursued by the Nazis. They exterminated tens of thousands of disabled people, having designated them 'life unworthy of life'. This programme served as the experimental forerunner for the racial genocide of Jews and other 'non-Aryan' groups (Weale 2001).

Revulsion at the Nazi Holocaust made eugenic arguments anathema for a time after the Second World War, but the rise of modern genetics helped put it back on the agenda. One argument used by modern-day eugenicists to distance themselves from policies and practices of previous eras is that it was politicians, not scientists, who were responsible for the mass murder of disabled people. In this view, the abuses of the Nazis are put down to 'one man and his odious politics' (Kealey 2000: 7). From this perspective eugenics is a 'benign' science and it is the political context that explains its oppressive use. This is questionable however. The overwhelming evidence is that it was medical scientists who carried out the euthanasia programme in Nazi Germany. Furthermore, the social and political context which allowed the Nazi euthanasia policy to function with little opposition was one generated by influential scientists expounding negative views of disability and disabled people (Russell 1998). Such negativity persists, and draws new strength from the ideas of sociobiology and evolutionary psychology. Like eugenics before them, these theories walk the thin line between scientific theory and social ideology. But let us now examine the way genetic medicine is actually approaching disability.

The curative approach proposes that in mapping the human genome and 'cracking the genetic code' we shall be able to manipulate genes to achieve therapeutic ends, including the 'curing' of genetic disease and impairment. However, there are serious question marks emerging over the capacity of genetic science to actually deliver on this promise. Kevles (1999: 298) points out that, 'like intelligence, most human characteristics are polygenic, and therefore not even genetically understood, let alone subject to manipulation'. Genetics based on such a determinist paradigm appears to have sold itself on the promise of what Ho (1999: 48) calls a 'science that fails the reality test'. Thus the preventive approach, using prenatal screening (PNS) has taken precedence. Like the science, the ethics and politics here are complex however. This was revealed in a RADAR survey which canvassed the views of disabled people and their families about genetic medicine (Royal Association for Disability and Rehabilitation (RADAR) 1999). Some who were opposed to abortion generally, for instance, argued that it might be justifiable in the case of impairment detected by PNS procedures. Others who expressed disquiet about PNS were nonetheless anxious that such disquiet should not be used to challenge a women's right to choose abortion. The complex interplay between the issues of abortion and PNS has been identified as an issue, therefore, which requires caution and sensitivity (Shakespeare 1999).

The main fear expressed in the RADAR survey, however, was that the increased use of PNS will be used to question the quality of life of disabled people. There is a fear that the selection process in PNS will be used to promote discrimination on the basis of genetic make-up. There is also the belief that the claim of medicine to be offering parents a choice is disingenuous given the negativity with which disability is often perceived by the medical profession, and the pressure which is consequently applied to parents to abort in the event of a positive test. This is a point raised by the Down's Syndrome Association in its response to the assertion by a leading embryologist that PNS will make it a 'sin' for parents to have a disabled child (Rogers 1999). The high moral tone taken here is reminiscent of Social Darwinist eugenicists in the early twentieth century, and is a good example of the way in which scientific opinion shapes the social context in which disability exists. The impact of such views, from such sources, is to create a hostile social environment for, and to undermine the cultural status of, disabled people (Wolbring 2001).

The negative view of disability widely held in western culture is based, it is currently being argued, on two erroneous assumptions. First, that disability equals a tragic and disrupted state, and second, that it is automatically associated with a life of isolation, poverty and powerlessness (Asch 2001). The origin of these views lies primarily in medical conceptions of disability as equivalent to disease and a departure from a desired state of 'health'. Disability is, according to these assumptions, something that no one in their right mind would choose for themselves or their child, and it is indeed a condition from which one should actively want to escape. This logic underpins medical, legal and bioethical support for euthanasia of disabled adults, infants and foetuses. It is this perspective that has been challenged most strongly by the disability rights movement. They have argued that such a view ignores crucial social dimensions of disability, and particularly the fact that, if disabled people do indeed live lives characterized by isolation, poverty and powerlessness, then that is more to do with political, economic and cultural than biological factors (Morris 1991). Disabled people may well be driven to a despair that makes them wish to end their own lives, not as a result of anything inherent in their biological or genetic make-up, but as a result of social discrimination, prejudice and inadequate, inappropriate and oppressive service systems. Let us now look at this issue in relation to Huntington's disease, which is a rare genetic condition.

Questions for discussion

1 How might present-day genetic scientists defend themselves against accusations of resurrecting 'old style' eugenics?
2 Is the attempt to eradicate impairment using genetic approaches realistic?
3 What effect might the widespread use of prenatal screening have for disabled people in society?

Coping with genetic impairment: Huntington's disease

My source for this case study is Joanne, a person with wide experience of and involvement with Huntington's disease, in both a personal and professional capacity. As such she has been particularly well placed to observe the interface between society, human services and people with Huntington's disease. Joanne is a false name used to maintain anonymity.

Huntington's disease is a so-called 'single gene' condition. The name comes from George Huntington, a doctor who described a collection of symptoms and characteristics which includes progressive motor and cognitive impairment and personality changes. In the latter stages physical and cognitive impairment become progressively more profound, culminating in death. During the 10–20 years of its usual duration, between 20 per cent and 30 per cent of brain weight is lost, and it has been described as 'programmed brain death' (Rasko and Downes 1995: 240). Average age of onset is 38, although it varies between 25 and 70. Onset below that age is rare, although Joanne suggests it is commoner than believed, but is often missed, or mistaken for other things, including delinquency.

A good deal of Joanne's account of the issues facing people with Huntington's disease related to testing for the presence of the indicative genetic marker. This was identified in 1993, and the following year saw the development of a test to identify it. The presence of the genetic marker is a 100 per cent certain indicator that the individual will be affected, although there is no way of predicting when. Prenatal screening is available from ten weeks, with the same pressures to abort in the case of a positive test that have been noted elsewhere, being apparent in Joanne's experience. Otherwise testing will usually be performed only on adults over the age of 18, it being argued that children are not able to handle diagnosis.

In the case of adults there are frequently waiting periods of months which, Joanne relates, are highly stressful. Either a neurologist or a psychiatrist usually oversees the procedure. This reflects, in Joanne's view, an ambiguity in the medical response to the condition. There is some controversy as to whether Huntington's disease should be treated as an irreversible degenerative neurological condition, or a psychiatric condition managed by psychoactive medications and psychological support. This situation is exacerbated in cases where diagnosis has not been confirmed, but an individual is instead referred to psychiatric services for aggressive behaviour. Aggression is, in Joanne's experience, one of the early symptoms of brain changes produced by the condition, and is frequently not recognized for what it is. Joanne relates many experiences of individuals who fall foul of the law, and whose family life and social networks are severely disrupted before diagnosis is made.

The development of testing was, in Joanne's view, a positive thing. Most people in her experience want to know in order to be able to shape their lives, and also the lives of their families. The issues and experiences surrounding testing are highly complex and varied however. Many people have, for instance, experienced parents whose personality changes and aggression have shaped their views negatively. They argue that a positive test should result either in a decision to abort, or not to have children, on the grounds that we should not put someone through this experience if we do not have to. Others argue that, even with a positive test, quality of life is what matters, and that it should still be possible to live a happy and fulfilling life up to, and even during the onset and progression of impairment.

Joanne was quite scathing about claims of possible cures. The term she used to describe this was 'selling dreams'. In particular, she argued that this emphasis in thinking diverts funds away from research into other responses to Huntington's disease, particularly supporting individuals and their families attempting to live with its effects.

Support services for people and families living with Huntington's disease are, in Joanne's words 'appalling'. Services seem to be effectively immobilized by a kind of 'therapeutic nihilism'. Once a positive test result is received service input seems to evaporate. Often, no professional group or agency appears willing to take responsibility, with the result that support is often patchy, inconsistent and sometimes, absent altogether. This picture appears to be particularly true for those in the early stages of the disease. In Joanne's experience, the behavioural problems in this phase are often more problematic and demanding than the physiological impairments which follow, and yet it is only when the physical impairment manifests itself that support is given, and this is often barely sufficient. The picture painted here suggests that the negative medical prognosis attached to people with Huntington's disease results in them and their families virtually being 'written off'. Joanne recalls being told by one doctor 'What do you expect? They've got Huntington's disease!'

It appears then that disabled people's fears about the negative impact of genetic testing and diagnosis on their quality of life are well founded. For people living with genetically related impairments that negative impact is already apparent. It also appears that the dominance of the bio-reductionist paradigm in health care leads to an overemphasis on high-tech genetic research at the expense of research into ways in which people and their families living with these conditions can be supported to achieve and maintain a good quality of life.

The experience of people with Huntington's disease, and conditions like it offers challenges to the disabled people's movement too. The social model of disability on which the movement has based its challenge to society about the nature of disability has challenged the view that impairment is necessarily 'tragic' in its effects and impact on people's lives (French and Swain 2002). As pointed out earlier, for many disabled people 'suffering' and 'tragedy' are the result of socially imposed barriers and prejudices rather than anything inherent in their biological make-up. I would argue that Joanne's account strongly suggests that degenerative conditions like Huntington's disease can have a personally tragic aspect that needs to be acknowledged in order to embrace the experience of people who live with them. To ignore this is to ignore people's lived experience, and thus to alienate them and render them irrelevant.

The actual benefits of genetic medicine for disabled people are, at least at present, and possibly for the foreseeable future, hard to see. The main effect has been to resurrect, and give new sophistication and moral authority to the eugenic project that has always simmered just below the surface of medical science's view of disability. Perhaps the best response to this perspective is the promotion of an 'ecological' view of disability which places it at the heart of the social world where it is actually experienced by people in their relationships and interactions with other people and the material environment, rather than maintaining it as purely the concern of biomedicine and its obsession with seeking cures. Disability, genetically related or otherwise, is in this view, not so much an aberration to be eradicated, but a part of the diversity of the human condition. Like our genes, it is actually part of our individual and collective human heritage.

Questions for discussion

1 Why might people living with the risk of developing Huntington's disease prefer to know for certain if they will develop it?
2 How might services for people with Huntington's disease be organized to better support them and their families?
3 Is it better to spend money on looking for cures for genetic disease, or to spend it helping people live with it?

Debate activity

Debate the proposition: Life is always worth living whatever the level of impairment. The following quotations may provide you with a starting point:

> Selective abortion is morally problematic . . . First selective abortion expresses negative or discriminatory attitudes not merely about a disabling trait, but about those who carry it. Second it signals an intolerance of diversity not merely in the society but in the family, and ultimately it could harm parental attitudes towards children.
>
> (Parens and Asch 2000: 13)

The background to my decision is also my belief that, all other things equal, disability (specifically, a disability for which I would consider an abortion) would make life more difficult for my child, my family and me. This is not the same thing as saying it would be an overwhelming burden or make a fulfilling life impossible. It does not mean that my child, my family or I could not handle the difficulties. It means only that *if I have a choice,* I would prefer to avoid them for all of our sakes. And I believe I do have a choice.

(Baily 2000: 67, emphasis in original)

Further reading

Asch, A. (2001) Disability, bioethics and human rights, in G.L. Albrecht, K.D. Seelman and M. Bury (eds) *Handbook of Disability Studies.* London: Sage.

Bailey, R. (1996) Prenatal testing and the prevention of impairment: a woman's right to choose? in J. Morris (ed.) *Encounters with Strangers: Feminism and Disability.* London: The Women's Press.

Parens, E. and Asch, A. (eds) (2000) *Prenatal Testing and Disability Rights.* Washington, DC: Georgetown University Press.

Wolbring, G. (2001) Where do we draw the line? Surviving eugenics in a technological world, in M. Priestley (ed.) *Disability and the Life Course: Global Perspectives.* Cambridge: Cambridge University Press.

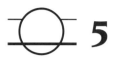 **5**

A dividing society?

With Ayesha Vernon

Questions of social divisions

I (JS) spent my youth in Beeston, Leeds and knew well the graveyard that is the setting for Tony Harrison's poem 'V', and these verses are, for me, an affective starting point for this chapter:

> These Vs are the versuses of life
> from LEEDS v. DERBY, Black/White
> and (as I've known to my cost) man v. wife,
> Communist v. Fascist, Left v. Right,
>
> Class v. class as bitter as before,
> the unending violence of US and THEM,
> personified in 1984
> by Coal Board MacGregor and the NUM,
>
> Hindu/Sikh, body/soul, heart v. mind,
> East/West, male/female, and the ground
> these fixtures are fought out on 's Man, resigned
> to hope from his future what his past never found.

> (Harrison 1987)

This chapter explores the 'versuses of life'. It is about our differences but also our commonalities, or 'social divisions'. The notion of social divisions is broad and is associated with other concepts in social theory, including hierarchies, equality/inequality, culture, poverty and identity. In particular we focus on that fact that we all have multiple possible identities, whether or not we embrace them: male/female, Black/white, young/old, heterosexual/homosexual and so on. The second section of the chapters picks up issues of multiple identity, particularly being Black, disabled and a woman. The case study is of the educational experiences of three Black disabled women.

Payne (2000: 1) claims that the idea of social divisions is one of the most useful and powerful tools available in understanding ourselves, society and why society operates as it does. Identity is a central concept in relation to social divisions and has increasingly come to prominence in areas of inquiry across the social sciences (Hetherington 1998). Our sense of who we are, our own identity in relation (sometimes 'versus') the identity of others is part and parcel of our lived experience and interwoven, and created within, our interactions with others. Our sense of who we are is linked, for instance, to our awareness of our identities as women or as men. Both gender and sexuality play a significant role in our understanding of identity, but, of course, what it means to be a man or woman also depends on the society we live in. Identity is at the interface between the personal, that is thoughts, feelings, personal histories, and the social, that is the societies in which we live and the social, cultural and economic factors which shape experience and make it possible for people to take up some identities and render others inaccessible or impossible (Woodward 2000: 18).

Questions of identity, then, take analysis into the political arena. Jenkins (1996) writes of resistance as potent affirmation of group identity:

> Struggles for a different allocation of resources and resistance to categorisation are one and the same thing . . . Whether or not there is an explicit call to arms in these terms, something that can be called self-assertion – or 'human spirit' is at the core of resistance to domination . . . It is as intrinsic, and as necessary, to that social life as the socialising tyranny of categorisation.
>
> (Jenkins 1996: 175)

Similarly, Hetherington (1998) suggests that identity has become significant through resistance to dominance in unequal power relations:

> One of the main issues behind this interest in identity and in identity politics more generally has been the relationship between marginalisation and a politics of resistance, and affirmative, empowering choices of identity and a politics of difference.
>
> (Hetherington 1998: 21)

'Politics of difference' can divide society into opposing groups, into 'them and us' and 'self and other', and where there is difference there is the potential for institutionalized discrimination (Thompson 2001). That is the unfair or unequal treatment of individuals or groups which is built into institutional organizations, policies and practices at personal, environmental and structural levels (Swain et al. 1998). It is a process through which groups and individuals experience different forms of oppression, including racism, sexism, ageism, disablism and so on. To take gender as an example, Abbott (2000) demonstrates a whole range of gender inequalities in employment and pensions, state benefits, labour market access and the poverty experienced by lone parent families. Work plays a key role. Despite other changes in paid employment patterns, women's earnings are still substantially lower than men's (Hatt

2000). Domestic work, including unpaid caring work, remains devalued and predominantly 'women's work'. Thompson (2001) suggests that forms of oppression can impact on identity in a number of ways:

1 Alienation, isolation and marginalisation – social exclusion from full participation in society;
2 Economic position and life-chances;
3 Confidence, self-esteem and aspirations; and
4 Social aspirations, career opportunities and so on.

(Thompson 2001: 140)

Concern about identity is also concern about change: challenging social expectations about identity; establishing new identities; and transforming existing identities (Jenkins 1996). Since the 1950s, 'new social movements', including the women's movement, the Black Power movement and, of course, the disabled people's movement, have played a significant role in the politics of identity (see Chapter 14). They can be seen as collective endeavours to give voice to and affirm new identities. It is apparent that the more overt the discrimination and oppression that people experience, the more heightened their awareness and sense of vulnerability around that particular identity. Monks (1999) states:

> People who are socially excluded and oppressed, and who are often also defined as lacking qualities of a normative social being, may find solidarity in the shared experience of exclusion itself . . . The 'communities' which emerge may become politically active . . . Experience of the interdependence, mutuality and solidarity which arise from shared activities and communication is an important part of membership, even of direct political action.
>
> (Monks 1999: 71)

For many social scientists, on the other hand, the broad picture is one of fractured, fluid, multiple and contested identities. According to Bradley (1996: 23), for instance, people can draw their sense of identity from a broad range of sources, including class, gender, age, marital status, sexual preference, consumption patterns and, we would add, disability. Furthermore, identity is a matter of 'becoming' rather than simply 'being':

> Far from being eternally fixed in some essentialized past, they are subject to the continuous 'play' of history, culture and power . . . identities are the names we give to the different ways we are positioned by, and position ourselves within, the narratives of the past.
>
> (Hall 1990: 225)

In a context of diversity and fluidity, identity is contested within conflicts of interest and power inequalities. Williams (1996) shows how the commonality between women stressed by feminism in the 1970s has been challenged:

> Feminism based on Black, lesbian and disabled politics has pointed to the need to deconstruct the category of 'woman' in order to understand the

complex and inter-connected range of identities and subject positions through which women's experiences are constituted, as well as the ways these also change over time and place.

(Williams 1996: 69)

This is a feature of most social movements. It is perhaps ironic that the very context in which people can become united is also a context in which divisions are affirmed. Thus, as a Black feminist writer, Lorde (1984), has stated:

Somewhere on the edge of consciousness, there is what I call a *mythical norm* . . . this norm is usually defined as white, thin, male, young, hetero-sexual, Christian and financially secure. It is with this mythical norm that the trappings of power reside within this society. Those of us who stand outside that power often identify one way in which we are different, and we assume that to be the primary cause of all oppression, forgetting other distortions around difference, some of which we ourselves may be prac-tising.

(Lorde 1984: 37)

From this viewpoint, oppression becomes much more diffuse than the idea that there are people who are oppressed and there are others who oppress. It is possible to be both oppressed and oppressor.

Questions for discussion

1 Thinking of yourself, what would you say are the main determinants of your identity, however you would define it?
2 How have identities changed in western societies over the past, say, fifty years? Think particularly of gender identities, what it meant to be a man or a woman in Britain just after the Second World War and what it means now.
3 Do you recognize yourself as both oppressed and oppressor? With whom and why?

Disabled people and multiple discrimination

Begum (1994a) states:

The very nature of simultaneous oppression means that as Black Disabled men and women, and Black disabled lesbians and gay men we cannot identify a single source of oppression to reflect the reality of our lives. No meaningful analysis of multiple oppression can take place without an acknowledgement that Black disabled people are subject to simultaneous oppression and as a consequence of this we cannot simply prioritise one aspect of our oppression to the exclusion of others.

(Begum 1994a: 35)

Thus, as argued by Stuart (1993), Black disabled people are subjected to a unique form of institutional discrimination which is different from the sum of racism experienced as a Black person and disablism experienced as a disabled person. Their experiences 'isolate black disabled people and place them at the margins of the ethnic minority and disabled populations' (Stuart 1993: 95).

The possession of multiple penalties may exacerbate the experience of one penalty. For example, disabled women's experience of sexism is often exacerbated by the intersection of gender and disability (Lonsdale 1990; Lloyd 1992). There seems to be a proliferation of additive approaches, such as 'double disadvantage' and 'triple burden', to capture the experience of disabled people encountering a number of forms of oppression. However, additive approaches are far from adequate, particularly because no one experience of oppression is uniform or fixed. Disabled people who have multiple identities experience both multiple and 'simultaneous oppression' because oppression occurs singularly, multiply and simultaneously in their lives, the dynamics of which vary from day to day and from context to context. For example, there is no uniform experience of racism because it is constituted not only in terms of existing social divisions but by diverse ethnicities and identities. Miles (1989: 57) points out that 'what is a collective disadvantage is not necessarily an individual disadvantage and, similarly, the determinant of the collective disadvantage is not necessarily the determinant of the individual disadvantage.'

Bhavnani (1994) states:

> Black women's experience cannot always be assumed to be different from white women, black men or white men in all contexts. The interplay of factors such as 'race', gender, class, age and disability create a multiplicity of discrimination. These may, in some contexts, suggest similarities with, as well as differences between, white women and black and white men.
>
> (Bhavnani 1994: viii)

The experience of racism may certainly be modified or exacerbated by an individual's class position. On the axes of privilege–penalty (Hill-Collins 1990), social class is an important determinant of many critical factors. As class privilege increases, the effects of other penalties are likely to decrease. Equally, lower social class positioning may exacerbate the effects of other penalties. Moreover, disablism and racism significantly lessen the chances of disabled people and Black and ethnic minority people progressing higher up the social class ladder, a fact evident in their high unemployment rate as well as their concentration in low paid and low skilled jobs (Schriner 2001). Nevertheless, not all disabled people or Black and ethnic minority people are in the same social class position and, in this complex picture, it can be that disability lessens the effects of other forms of oppression, such as sexism.

The multiple oppression faced by disabled people from Black and ethnic minority communities manifests itself in many ways in day-to-day living. The evidence relating to this particular group is sparse but points to major barriers at all levels of institutional discrimination. Discrimination within the provision of services has received particular attention, despite being denied and rationalized through myths that, for instance, Black families prefer 'to look after their own' (Baxter 1995). Though the literature documenting the views of Black disabled people is sparse, it consistently speaks to experiences of segregation and marginalization within services. Summarizing the evidence from several studies, Butt and Mirza (1996) state:

> The fact that major surveys of the experience of disability persist in hardly mentioning the experience of black disabled people should not deter us from appreciating the messages that emerge from existing work. Racism, sexism and disablism intermingle to amplify the need for supportive social care. However these same factors sometimes mean that black disabled people and their carers get a less than adequate service.
>
> (Butt and Mirza 1996: 94)

In their study of young Black disabled people's experiences and views, Bignall and Butt (2000) conclude:

> Our interviews revealed that most of these young people did not have the relevant information to help them achieve independence. Hardly any knew of new provisions, such as Direct Payments, which would help with independent living. Most people did not know where to get help or information they wanted, for example, to move into their own place or go to university.
>
> (Bignall and Butt 2000: 49)

Language is often seen as the main barrier to effective service provision. It is, therefore, assumed that an adequate supply of leaflets and interpreters in appropriate languages would solve the problem. However, communication consists of more than language skills and literacy. Research by Banton and Hirsch (2000) again bears out the findings of previous research. They state:

> Communication problems are identified in all work in this area. Such problems are partly to do with language differences, but also arise from the separate lives led by different ethnic groups in our society and the consequent unlikely coincidence of communications about services arising through informal contacts.
>
> (Banton and Hirsch 2000: 32)

Finally, perhaps the most consistent recommendation from research has been the necessity for the direct involvement of disabled clients, including Black disabled clients, in the planning of services (Butt and Box 1997). Again this needs to be understood within the context of multiple discrimination. Concluding their study with Asian deaf young people and their families, Jones et al. (2001) state:

> identities are not closely tied to single issues and young people and their families simultaneously held on to different identity claims. To this

extent, it is not a question of forsaking one claim for another and choosing, for instance, 'deafness' over 'ethnicity', but to negotiate the space to be deaf and other things as well. It is only through addressing these tensions that services will adequately respond to the needs of Asian deaf people and their families.

(Jones et al. 2001: 68)

The possibility of fragmentation within the disabled people's movement has been a recurring concern. Monks (1999), for instance, claims that:

By the early 1990s there was undeniable differentiation of the movement motivated by claims of *particular* experience of disablement. A current major dilemma for the movement, then, lies in the membership's recognition of peculiarities of experience being coupled with a commitment to collective political action.

(Monks 1999: 75, emphasis in original)

Morris (1991: 12) writes that 'Black disabled people and disabled gay men and lesbians express their particular concerns in particular contexts . . . such groups should not be treated as an "added on" optional extra to a more general analysis of disability.'

This fragmentation is potentially limitless with the interaction of different social divisions. In the 1990s, for instance, a number of groups have emerged to address a variety of concerns of minority ethnic disabled people. For instance:

Some groups consisted of Deaf people who had united on the basis of their 'blackness', while others targeted Deaf people who belonged to a particular ethnic group or had a particular religious affiliation. There were also groups which were exclusively for Deaf Asian women.

(Ahmad et al. 2000: 73)

REGARD is a campaigning organization of disabled lesbians and gay men established to address the heterosexism that exists within the disabled people's movement and society generally. The research by Gillespie-Sells et al. (1998) suggests that the establishment of a collective and democratic voice of disabled lesbians and gay men is, however, problematic:

Discussion with REGARD revealed a reluctance on behalf of Black disabled lesbians to 'come out' and be identified. The reason put forward was homophobia in the disability community . . . There were also problems of anti-lesbianism within families and minority ethnic communities in addition there was a lack of support to tackle the hostility that asserting their sexuality aroused.

(Gillespie-Sells et al. 1998: 62)

Another more recent addition to the list of groups with fragmented identities whose interests are not fully addressed by single issue movements is disabled refugees and asylum seekers who 'constitute one of the most disadvantaged groups within our society' (Roberts 2000: 945). Disabled refugees and asylum seekers are 'lost in the system' because both 'the disability movement and the refugee community focus their attention . . . on issues affecting the majority of their populations and fail to engage adequately with issues which affect a small minority' (Roberts 2000: 945).

Questions for discussion

1 In what ways might disabled people's experiences of discrimination differ, depending on multiple identities, and in what ways might their experiences be the same?
2 Is the notion that some disabled people are more oppressed than other disabled people a potentially useful idea? Why, or if not why not?
3 Can such a diverse group as disabled people have sufficient commonalities of experience to be unified within a disabled people's movement? If so, how?

A childhood apart

This case study uses published accounts by three Black, disabled women, who all went to special schools, to explore their educational experiences (Nasa Begum, Ayesha Vernon and Angela Smith). Nasa Begum, who went to a day school for physically disabled children, between the 1950s and 1960s, spoke of the verbal bullying she received from white pupils:

> As a child it was hard for me to accept that there were two distinct ways I was different from the majority, not like the people I saw on the TV, in the comics and books I read. At school everyone had some form of disability so no one was picked on just for that. But disabled kids are just like everyone else and they would tease out and pick on anyone who was different. I had never thought about it before I started school but I soon learned what it meant to be black in a predominantly white establishment. I used to get very upset at the relentless name-calling, 'blackie', 'nigger', 'paki', but grassing on anyone was not on so I had to learn to live with it.
>
> (Begum 1994b: 49)

Ayesha Vernon had similar experiences between the 1970s and early 1980s:

> I could only speak very basic English. Communication was very difficult, I was the only Asian girl there. I had kids laughing at my English and I had difficulty making them understand what I wanted. Culturally it was very different. I ate Asian food. I wore Asian clothes. I had been brought up to be a very strict Muslim. I learned very quickly that I had to adapt,

I had to change otherwise it wasn't going to work, I wasn't going to be accepted and I would be isolated.

(Vernon quoted in French et al. 1997: 24)

Angela Smith recalls how her personal care needs were not met at her special residential school, in the 1970s, and the consequences of this for her well-being and self-esteem:

In the case of my hair care, the house parents were ignorant as to how to comb and plait my hair. They would wash it and leave it. Each time I returned home I had to spend a day having my hair painfully detangled. My Mum tried to overcome this problem by straightening my hair. This involved putting oils in my hair. White people tend to associate greasy hair with dirty hair. Consequently, when I returned from home with my hair straightened, my house parents would wrongly assume that my hair was dirty and wash it out . . . I started to resent being Black.

(Smith 1994: 128)

She goes on to say:

There was a brief period when there was an Afro Caribbean student, on placement, in the school for a term. For obvious reasons she took an interest in myself and another African Caribbean pupil. The first thing she did was to sort out our matted, tangled hair and moisturize our dry, cracked skin. My self-esteem shot up by about 110%.

(Smith 1994: 130)

Meeting other Black, disabled people could also be very important. Nasa Begum (1994b) writes:

There was only one other Asian girl at my school and I always admired her. She had a wonderful dress sense and beautiful long black hair which fell from her shoulders right down to the base of her spine . . . She was the only black role model that I had. Her culture was very different from mine and her experience of family life was not the same, but the fact that she was at my school was important for me. Until I met her, I had never seen another Asian person with a disability and I was proud to be considered like her.

(Begum 1994b: 49–50)

Clothes, food and other basic aspects of their cultural heritage were ignored by the schools. Nasa Begum talks of the problems she experienced with dress:

My Mum used to sew me the Salwar Kamiz, matching silk dresses and trousers, like she did for my sisters, but they just attracted further derogatory remarks at school until I begged her to let me stop wearing them. Eventually she relented and bought me Western-style trousers and dresses. Even this didn't help because my culture said that girls should wear both trousers and dresses but according to my school friends this was the pits of fashion. I ended up feeling uncomfortable in the clothes I wore at school and at home and I tried to solve this dilemma by wearing

Western clothes at school and changing immediately I returned. For about fifteen years I did not allow white people to see me in Salwar Kamiz.

Begum (1994b: 49)

Angela Smith had similar experiences:

The social consequences of being in a culturally inappropriate environment had a detrimental effect emotionally . . . All of the house parents were white. My dietary needs were never considered, it was assumed that I ate English food. I remember that I used to get cravings for some home cooked West Indian cooking.

(Smith 1994: 128)

The women also studied a curriculum that did not take their culture into account. Angela Smith recalled:

My education was eurocentric. The curriculum consisted of the three 'R's' plus history, geography, science, biology and home economics. These were all taught from a European perspective. All the innovations and revolutions that took place were brought about by white people . . . I often felt a sense of being disconnected. I would think to myself, where were my ancestors; what were they doing while Henry VIII was collecting the heads of his wives?

Smith (1994: 127)

Disabled people who have been sent away to boarding schools often remark on the estrangement this causes from their families. Eve (in French 1996), for example, recalls:

I didn't seem to feel like one of the family. I felt detached from them quite early on. I don't see a lot of my family now and I think the early separation is probably why. I remember my parents saying, a long time afterwards, that I was very withdrawn when they first took me out for a visiting day and that I didn't say anything to them unless they spoke to me first.

(quoted in French 1996: 20)

For Black disabled people, however, this can be more profound as they are likely to experience separation from their entire culture. Angela Smith writes:

I became aware that I was growing apart from my family . . . This was not because of my disability. It was because I had spent a large proportion of my childhood in a different environment. It was a predominantly white middle class setting. I had a different experience of childhood and adolescence from my brothers and sisters. I wanted to be able to relate to things that they were interested in. For example, Black youth culture, music clubs, clothes, ideas and jargon. I could not relate to any of it. I had even lost my appetite for some Caribbean dishes. It felt as though I was a stranger in my own culture.

(Smith 1994: 132–3)

Questions for discussion

1 Nasa Begum, Ayesha Vernon and Angela Smith were looking back to their time at special school. Do you think anything has changed in recent years? If so what changes do you think have been made?
2 How might experiences at school affect the long-term identity of Black disabled women?
3 Angela Smith mentions that the curriculum she studied was Euro-centric. How far does the school curriculum address issues of race, culture and disability today?

Debate activity

Debate the proposition: Unity in the disabled people's movement is crucial to the elimination of oppression faced by disabled people. The following quotations may provide you with a starting point.

I am of the belief that black disabled people share a lot in common with white disabled people. We have lots of issues in common but we cannot ignore the fact that to a very large extent there still is that added element of racism that we have to encounter as black people. I didn't think that the white disability movement was taking that on board.

(Hill in Campbell and Oliver 1996: 132)

Disabled people have no choice but to attempt to build a better world because it is impossible to have a vision of inclusionary capi-talism: we all need a world where impairment is valued and cele-brated and all disabling barriers are eradicated. Such a world would be inclusionary for all.

(Oliver and Barnes 1998: 62)

Further reading

Ahmad, W.I.U. (ed.) (2000) *Ethnicity, Disability and Chronic Illness*. Buckingham: Open University Press.
Begum, N., Hill, M. and Stevens, A. (eds) (1994) *Reflections: Views of Black Disabled People on their Lives and Community Care*. London: Central Council for Education and Train-ing in Social Work.
Payne, G. (ed.) (2000) *Social Divisions*. London: Macmillan Press.
Thompson, N. (2001) *Anti-Discriminatory Practice*, 3rd edn. Basingstoke: Palgrave.

6

Celebrating difference?

Being different

This chapter explores the impact on people's lives of being labelled 'different'. Being different can incur admiration and praise but more often it leads to prejudice, discrimination and oppression. Oppressed people are, however, increasingly affirming their identity and insisting that their difference is a cause for celebration. The first section of this chapter explores the impact of being negatively labelled on various groups within society and how they have affirmed and celebrated their identity; women who choose to be childless will be the main example. The second section examines the issue of 'difference' in the lives of disabled people and the development of the affirmative model of disability. The third section of the chapter focuses on the disability arts movement where alternative understandings of both disability and impairment have been promoted.

Many people are perceived to be tragic, dangerous, inferior or less than human because they do not conform to societal norms. These norms change with social, economic and political circumstances so our perceptions of others vary over time and across cultures. Gay men in Britain, for example, were until the 1967 Sex Offenders Act regarded as criminal and cast into jail for their sexual activities. Later they were given an illness label and 'treated' by psychiatrists who attempted to 'cure' them. More recently a fragile acceptance of their lifestyle has emerged although enormous prejudice still exists which is reflected in legislation and social policy. It is, for example, still very difficult for gay couples to adopt a child and gay partnerships are not given the same legal or social status as heterosexual marriage.

In recent years lesbians and gay men have 'come out', have rejected the labels imposed on them and have celebrated their difference by establishing organizations such as Gay Pride. They have asserted a positive identity which has counteracted the negative identity imposed on them by others and which they may, in part, have internalized themselves.

Another group who are stigmatized in most societies are women who choose not to have children, though in many developing countries no choice exists (Foreman 1999a). Such women are often regarded as selfish, hedonistic, feckless, child-hating and unfulfilled (Bartlett 1994; Safer 1996; McAllister with Clarke 1998). Many of the women whom Bartlett interviewed spoke of negative attitudes, pressure to become parents from family and friends and an erosion of self-esteem. One woman said, 'Often in a social situation I feel the odd one out . . . you're a woman, you don't marry, and you don't have children as well. That means I'm a non-person' (Bartlett 1994: 25). Similarly a woman interviewed by Safer (1996: 46), referring to family gatherings, said, 'I'm the only one there without a child so they think of me as less than evolved. There's a certain hush when people say, "she doesn't have children" – they always bring up a person they know who had a child in her late forties. People talk as if you had a fatal disease.'

Childless women are, however, beginning to speak out about the way they view motherhood. Safer (1996) openly admits that:

> in some essential ways I seemed temperamentally unsuited for the job. As heretical as it was to admit it, I realised that having a child of my own would force me to spend a great deal of time doing things I disliked . . . I recoiled at the chaos and limitations a baby would bring.
>
> (Safer 1996: 20)

Such is the stigma attached to women who choose to be childless that in 1978 the British Organization of Non-Parents (BON) was founded. The organization asserts that non-parents are 'different but equal' and states that:

> BON has been founded on the premise that the cultural and media bias against those without children must be redressed, and the organization seeks to stress that a life without children can be perfectly rewarding and fulfilling for those who choose it . . . The media and especially advertising constantly push the message that having children is fun, natural and necessary. There is a strong implication that if you do not conform there is something WRONG with you . . . BON gives you the opportunity to know that you are not unique or 'freakish' and a chance to hear from or speak to others who feel the same.
>
> (BON undated pamphlet)

BON has provided support and solidarity to many elective non-parents and has helped them to resist pressure, to feel valued and to assert and maintain a positive self-identity.

The choices open to women have greatly increased in western society since the early 1950s. This has resulted from the development of contraception and greater gender equality, for example in education, employment and the law. These changes have reduced the dependence of women on men and have opened up lifestyles which were previously unobtainable and where marriage and family are no longer central. The spearhead for most of these changes has been the women's movement which has a long history predating the mid-nineteenth century when women campaigned for the vote. More recent feminist analyses view motherhood as an oppressive institution that is dominated by men. Lawler (1996) states that

> engaging in maternal work, which is only one, temporary aspect of a woman's life, has come to be defined as the whole of her identity . . . Nurturance, patience and the rest are not valued (or paid) because it is considered 'only natural' that women should care selflessly and unconditionally not only for children but for adult men also . . . Even if women do not become mothers they cannot escape the oppressiveness of the institution of motherhood . . . If women do not bear children then their childlessness is what defines them.
>
> (Lawler 1996: 154–5)

It has to be said, however, that the pressure to have children applies only to *some* women. Single women, lesbians and disabled women, for example, are often regarded as unfit to be mothers and can find themselves subjected to disapproval when they want to have children.

There are many other groups within society who are devalued including old people, people from ethnic minorities and those who are labelled mentally ill. Almost without exception the response to oppression is self-organization as a means of fighting back. The Black Civil Rights Movement, Mad Pride and the Association of Retired and Persons over 50 are all examples of organizations that challenge oppression at both a personal and political level.

Questions for discussion

1 Have you ever been labelled negatively? How, if at all, did you reduce the impact of it?
2 How may group identity change the feelings and behaviour of people who are negatively labelled?
3 How may social, economic, cultural and political changes impact (for better or worse) on people who are negatively labelled?

Celebrating disability and impairment

Throughout history and in most cultures disabled people have been viewed as inferior, dangerous, tragic, pathetic and not quite human. They have been kept apart from other people by the practice of institutionalization and by hostile attitudes and an inaccessible environment (Hughes 1998). Such are the negative presumptions held about impairment and disability, that the abortion of impaired foetuses is barely challenged (Parens and Asch 2000) and compulsory sterilization of people with learning difficulties has been widely practised in many parts of the world (Park and Radford 1999).

The erroneous idea that disabled people cannot contribute to society, or enjoy an adequate quality of life, lies at the heart of this response. The problems that disabled people experience are seen to result from impairment rather than the failure of society to meet that person's needs in terms of appropriate human help and accessibility. Furthermore people who acquire an impairment are assumed to suffer feelings of loss from which there will be no gain and from which they will never completely recover. Many disabled people have internalized these ideas resulting in a negative self-image for, as Linton (1998b: 152) points out, 'Disabled people and nondisabled people have both been schooled in the same ableist discourse.' Similarly Morris (1991) states:

> Most of the people we have dealings with, including our most intimate relationships, are not like us. It is therefore very difficult for us to recognise and challenge the values and judgements that are applied to us and our lives. Our ideas about disability and about ourselves are generally formed by those who are not disabled.
>
> (Morris 1991: 37)

Disabled people who view their impairments as positive or neutral have found it difficult or impossible to convince non-disabled people that this is the case (Linton 1998a). Talking of Helen Keller, Crow (2000: 854) states that 'It seemed that she could never fully satisfy people's curiosity for details nor could she reassure them entirely that she was content herself. When the non-disabled world feted her courage, for Helen, her impairments were a natural, largely neutral condition.' Similarly Kent (2000) writes:

> I will always believe that blindness is a neutral trait, neither to be prized nor shunned. Very few people including those dearest to me share that conviction . . . I feel that I have failed them when I run into jarring reminders that I have not changed their perspective. In those crushing moments I fear that I am not really accepted after all.
>
> (Kent 2000: 62)

In recent years disabled people have formed a vibrant international movement which has challenged the disabling physical and social environment in which they are compelled to live. A central aim of the disabled people movement has been to change the definition of disability from one of helplessness and tragedy, brought about by impairment, to one of civil rights and equality where disabling barriers are believed to be the cause of disability.

The affirmative model of disability (Swain and French 2000) extends the social model by focusing on the benefits and positive aspects of being disabled and having an impairment. This is a direct challenge to the tragedy model and is likely to be interpreted as an expression of bravery or simply ignored. The writings and experiences of disabled people demonstrate, however, that, far from being tragic, being disabled can have benefits. If, for example, a person has sufficient resources, giving up paid employment and pursuing interests and hobbies, following an accident, may enhance that person's life. Similarly, disabled people sometimes find that they can escape class oppression, abuse or neglect by virtue of being disabled. Martha, a Malaysian woman with a visual impairment whom we interviewed, was separated from a poor and neglectful family and sent to a special school at the age of 5. She said:

> I got a better education that any of them [siblings] and much better health care too. We had regular inoculations and regular medical and dental checks.

She subsequently went to university and qualified as a teacher which none of her brothers or sisters achieved. Similarly, the deaf children on Martha's Vineyard (an island off the east coast of the USA which had a high incidence of inherited deafness) were the only ones to receive an education (Groce 1985). Many children who were sent to 'open air' schools, because of conditions such as asthma and tuberculosis, escaped appalling poverty. Peter Holmes recalled:

> My first impression at the age of seven or eight was its vastness. Previously all I had ever seen was factories, terraced houses and bomb-sites. To a child like myself it was magnificent. The countryside and woods were overwhelming and very beautiful and the air so sweet . . . We would walk through the woods and visit farms seeing animals and flowers and trees that most of us had only ever seen in books . . . The food was very good. We also had indoor toilets and bathrooms, something we did not have at home, and real toilet paper – not newspaper.
>
> (quoted in Wilmot and Saul 1998: 257)

A further way in which disability and impairment may be perceived as beneficial to some disabled people is that society's expectations and requirements are more difficult to satisfy and may, therefore, be legitimately avoided. A disabled man quoted by Shakespeare et al. (1996: 81) said, 'I am never going to be able to conform to society's requirements and I am thrilled because I am blissfully released from all that crap. That's the liberation of disfigurement.'

Young people (particularly women) are frequently under pressure to form heterosexual relationships, to marry and have children. These expectations are not applied so readily to disabled people who may, indeed, be viewed as asexual. Although this has the potential to cause a great deal of anxiety and pain, some disabled people can see its advantages. As Vasey (1992b: 74) says, 'We are not usually snapped up in the flower of youth for our domestic and child rearing skills, or for our decorative value, so we do not have to spend years disentangling ourselves from wearisome relationships as is the case with many non-disabled women.'

Although it is more difficult for disabled people to form sexual relationships, because of disabling environmental and social barriers, when they do any limitations imposed by impairment may, paradoxically, lead to advantages. Shakespeare et al. (1996: 106), who interviewed disabled people about their sexuality and sexual relationships remark that, 'Because disabled people are not able to make love in a straight forward manner, or in a conventional position, they were impelled to experiment and enjoyed a more interesting sexual life as a result.'

For some people who become disabled their lives change completely though not necessarily for the worse. A woman quoted by Morris (1989) states:

> As a result of becoming paralysed life has changed completely. Before my accident it seemed as if I was set to spend the rest of my life as a religious sister, but I was not solemnly professed so was not accepted back into the order. Instead I am now very happily married with a home of my own.
>
> (Morris 1989: 120)

Basnett (2001), a disabled doctor, states:

> I was horrified by what I imagined to be the experience of disabled people, which I encountered in my practice. Now 15 years after becoming disabled, I find myself completely at home with the concept, of effectively being me! . . . Now I know that my assessment of the potential quality of life of severely disabled people was clearly flawed.
>
> (Basnett 2001: 453)

As for non-disabled people, the quality of life of disabled people depends on whether they can achieve a lifestyle of their choice. This, in turn, depends on their personal resources, the resources within society and their own unique situation. Morris (1993a) believes that the assumption that disabled people want to be other than who they are is one of the most oppressive experiences to which they are subjected.

The writings of disabled people demonstrate that being born with an impairment or becoming disabled later in life can give a perspective on life which is both interesting and affirmative and can be used positively. This is illustrated in the following quotations:

> A few years later, at my special school, I remember one of the care staff loudly telling me that I should never give up hope because one day doctors would find a cure for my affliction, and I loudly told her that I didn't want to be 'cured'. I remember this incident because of the utter disbelief this statement caused among all the non-disabled people present, and the delight this statement caused amongst all my disabled friends.
>
> (Mason 2000: 8)

> I cannot wish that I had never contracted ME, because it has made me a different person, a person I am glad to be, would not want to miss being and could not relinquish even if I were cured.
>
> (Wendell 1996: 83)

> I do not wish for a cure for Asperger's Syndrome. What I wish for is a cure for the common ill that pervades too many lives, the ill that makes people compare themselves to a normal that is measured in terms of perfect and absolute standards, most of which are impossible for anyone to reach.
>
> (Holliday Willey 1999: 96)

Some people who acquire an impairment do experience feelings of loss although this is by no means inevitable. John Hull (1991, 1997), for example, writes that he grieved for four and a half years over his loss of sight. His grieving process did, however, subside and being disabled has led him to write informative and penetrating books about the experience of blindness.

Nobody can accurately predict the amount of tragedy or happiness a person will experience in life – there are thousands of interacting variables and, in addition, there are numerous ways of viewing any situation – and yet people feel confident to make such predictions about disabled people without asking them or conceiving of a society where disabled people are accepted and included. The inherent assumption is that disabled people want to be other than as they are, even though this would mean a rejection of identity and self. For many disabled people the tragedy view of disability is in itself disabling. It denies their experiences of a disabling society, their enjoyment of life, and even their identity and self-awareness as disabled people.

Questions for discussion

1 Why is the tragedy model of disability so prevalent?
2 Why have disabled people rejected the tragedy model of disability?
3 What are the major ideas underpinning the affirmative model of disability and how, if at all, does it add to the social model of disability?

From tragedy to pride: disability arts

Disability arts is a relatively recent, though well-established, branch of the disabled people's movement. A wide variety of activities are encompassed within disability arts including theatre, dance, poetry, photography, comedy, music and visual art. Although disability arts is concerned with gaining access for disabled people to mainstream artistic facilities and opportunities, its main function is to communicate the distinctive history, skills, customs, experiences and concerns of disabled people, which many believe constitute a distinctive lifestyle and culture (Vasey 1992b). Disability arts gives disabled individuals the opportunity to express their views and experiences of impairment and disability which often run counter to mainstream stereotypes. A central feature of disability arts is, however, collective experience. Disabled people are increasingly coming together to help each other express themselves in art and to share information and ideas. Barnes et al. (1999) define disability arts as:

> the development of shared cultural meanings and the collective expression of the experience of disability and struggle. It entails using art to expose the discrimination and prejudice disabled people face and to generate group consciousness and solidarity. Disability cabarets can empower people in much the same way as going on a direct action demonstration.
>
> (Barnes et al. 1999: 205–6)

Disability arts is a political as well as an artistic endeavour. It involves making the implicit theories of disability explicit by exposing the derogatory nature of disablist images and stereotypes and challenging negative attitudes, discrimination and oppression. Through their art disabled people are promoting very different images of disability. Oliver and Barnes (1998) argue that disability arts produces, at one and the same time, a culture of resistance and celebration. Morrison and Finkelstein (1993: 27) state that, 'The arts can have a liberating effect on people . . . having someone on stage communicating ideas and feelings that an isolated disabled person never suspected were shared by others can be a turning point for many.'

The active participation of disabled people in disability arts does, in itself, combat images of passivity and dependence and can raise political awareness and self-esteem. As Corbett (1996) states:

> One of the distinctive features of this assertive energy, found in all groups that seek an identity which fosters their proud image, is in its focus on artistic expression. Whether it is in photography or art, sculpture or dance, acting or singing, disability arts has become a definite part of the new language of a political movement that seeks a wide audience and which supports diverse voices celebrating the joy of difference.
>
> (Corbett 1996: 25)

An example of a disability arts organization is DASh (Disability Arts in Shropshire). Ruth Kaye, a visually impaired writer and poet, is the chairperson of DASh and was interviewed for this chapter. Below is one of her poems which portrays her experience as a visually impaired person:

Seat

I asked for an empty seat,
She said 'Over there'
And waved her hand in the air, somewhere.
At a seat she could see –
Which meant
Nothing at all
To me.

So I faltered into empty space,
'No, not that way!'
I could hear the anger in her face
Curling to her feet
As she pinched me hard into my place,
Into that empty seat
And tidied me away
So I said
'Thank you'.

DASh was founded in 1992 as the Disability Arts Initiative. It has a wide range of funders including the Arts Council, District and County Councils of

Shropshire, the Regional Arts Lottery Programme and West Midland Arts. The members of DASh have a wide spectrum of impairments, including learning difficulties, and practise many art forms including photography, dance, drama, writing, video, embroidery, sculpture and woodwork. Since 1996 DASh has organized a disability arts festival every year where local and established artists from all disciplines, and from both inside and outside the region, perform their art. It also funds disabled people to train in mainstream organizations and has a year-round programme of workshops aimed at developing the skills of local disabled artists. DASh produces a monthly news-sheet which gives information about art events and job and training opportunities throughout the UK and abroad. One of DASh's current projects, which extends beyond the organization, is the production of a disability arts book on the theme of *Utopia*. It will feature many different art forms and will be launched at a disability arts exhibition in 2003.

An annual countrywide exhibition of commissioned work, the DASH-BASH, tours throughout the region and beyond helping to foster the skills of disabled artists and to develop new networks and audiences. DASh is also involved, through an initiative entitled Beyond the Ramp, in addressing access issues for disabled people in mainstream art. An important area of the organization's work is to provide a forum for social contact among disabled artists where they can share ideas and experiences. Ruth states that DASh 'is a very friendly, open, wide thinking, daring, adventurous and talented organisation.'

DASh gives disabled artists the opportunity to see and experience the work of others and to evaluate their own work. Some members of DASh make their living as artists while for others it is a hobby. Ruth, who has had a career in journalism, has written poetry since she was 11. She was always told that it was good, but DASh has given her extra confidence and has provided her with opportunities to publish and perform her work. Although members of DASh do not necessarily confine themselves to expressing ideas and experiences about disability, Ruth believes that disability always comes through in their art. She explains:

> When you're disabled everything you do has disability reflected in it. It has to because that's who you are, and art is always expressed from who you are. I know when I'm writing about something that is not meant to be about disability you can still feel it in there if you read it in a certain way. Our minds are set around disability and our work shows that.

There are no restrictions on how people choose to express themselves at DASh. Although the work of some artists may express anger at their situation as disabled people, Ruth is more concerned with finding commonalities and aiding people's understanding of disability by 'pricking something in their mind or heart.' In her poem, 'The Bucket', for example, the problem which is portrayed may or may not relate to disability:

The Bucket

1st   'My head is stuck in a bucket
       And I can't remove it.'

2nd   'Your head? Stuck? In a bucket?
       Well, can you prove it?'

1st   'Listen to the muffled echoes of my voice
       And hear the rattling tin.
       You must believe, you have no choice,
       It's a bucket that I'm in.

       Will you take it off for me?
       And let me reappear?
       I'm not complaining needlessly –
       It isn't nice in here.'

2nd   'Well how did the bucket get there?
       Did someone force you in?
       What makes you think that I should care
       If you are wrapped in tin?'

1st   'The bucket put itself on me
       Before I'd time to scream,
       I saw it come determinedly –
       But thought it was a dream.

       It was as if the bucket knew me
       And picked me from the crowd
       And now its fastened to me,
       Like some cold, metallic shroud.'

2nd   'Well, then, if the bucket needs you
       And knew your head was bare,
       I'm afraid I cannot please you,
       You'll have to stay in there.'

Disability arts is one of the powerful ways in which disabled people have expressed their positive identity and their personal and collective experience of impairment and disability. Disabled people are creating positive images of themselves and are demanding the right to be the way they are – to be equal but different.

Questions for discussion

1 Is disability arts a personal or a political activity?
2 How far does disability arts affirm and celebrate the experience of disability and impairment?
3 What impact might disability arts have on the majority perceptions of disabled people?

Debate activity

Debate the proposition: Far from being tragic, impairment and disability are a cause for celebration. The following quotations may provide you with a starting point.

> I can't imagine becoming hearing, I'd need a psychiatrist, I'd need a speech therapist, I'd need some new friends, I'd lose all my old friends, I'd lose my job . . . It really hits hearing people that a deaf person doesn't want to become hearing. I am what I am.
>
> (Shakespeare et al. 1996: 184)

> When I go out I don't know whether I'm passing someone I know or not, unless they speak to me. And I feel shut off a bit, I feel isolated by that. Because I used to go along that path and people used to say 'Hello, hello there' you know. Now I go passed and nobody . . . it's a feeling of isolation . . . I've lost all my social life. I've lost all that, apart from my family.
>
> (French et al. 1997: 38)

Further reading

Linton, S. (1998) *Claiming Disability: Knowledge and Identity*. New York: New York University Press.

Mason, M. (2000) *Incurably Human*. London: Working Press.

Morris, J. (1991) *Pride against Prejudice: Transforming Attitudes to Disability*. London: The Women's Press.

Swain, J. and French, S. (2000) Towards an affirmation model of disability, *Disability and Society*, 15(4): 569–82.

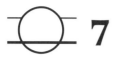 **7**

What's so good about independence?

What is independence?

This chapter concerns the meaning of independence in the lives of disabled people. Disabled people have argued that the tendency to define independence in narrow terms and the whole 'independence versus dependence' ideology has had an adverse effect on their quality of life. The chapter begins with a broad discussion of the meaning of independence in different cultures. It then examines how the notion of independence has oppressed disabled people and their struggle to expose the assumptions on which it is based. Finally the chapter highlights the policy of 'direct payment' which has helped some disabled people achieve independence on their own terms.

The word 'independence' has more than one meaning which can lead to great confusion. Perhaps the most prevalent definition concerns self-sufficiency. The *Collins School Dictionary* states: 'Someone who is independent does not need other people's help.' This simple definition is, however, flawed. We are all dependent on each other for at least some of our physical, social and emotional needs. As Parker (1993: 11) states, 'we rely on each other in a multitude of ways from the provision of the essentials of food, water and shelter to the complexities of feelings of self esteem.'

The *Collins Paperback English Dictionary* gives a more complex definition of independence, not only defining it as 'Capable of acting for oneself or on one's own' but as 'Free from control in judgement, action etc.'. Independence can, therefore, be defined in two main ways: our ability to look after ourselves without the help of others; and the control we are able to exercise over our lives whether or not we need assistance to do so.

The notion of independence in terms of self-sufficiency has been reinforced in British society in recent years by the political doctrine of individualism which can be defined as 'any set of ideas emphasising the importance of the individual and the individual's interests' (Marshall 1998: 304). The post-war

Labour government of Britain had a somewhat collectivist ideology and introduced various social benefits and services including family allowances and the
National Health Service (NHS). In the 1980s, however, Margaret Thatcher's
Conservative government cut public expenditure and emphasized 'self-help'
and individual enterprise. The political ideology thus shifted from collectivism
to individualism. As Margaret Thatcher pronounced in an interview in
Woman's Own magazine in October 1987:

> There is no such thing as society. There are individual men and women,
> and there are families. And no government can do anything except
> through people, and people must look to themselves first. It's our duty to
> look after ourselves and then, also to look after our neighbour.
>
> (cited in Hoggart 1995: 1)

In most countries of the world there are similar tensions between intervention
by the state and a belief in individual enterprise (Thomas 2000). All human
societies are characterized by interdependency, but some countries and
cultures are more oriented to collectivism than individualism. In some cultures
individuals are expected to put the good of the community above their own
wishes and interests. Religious values or bearing many children, for example,
may be deemed more important than individual wealth or personal achieve-
ments. Wirz and Hartley (1999) state that in the majority world, independence
may be an empty concept with interdependence being the key value.

In most countries there is a tension between collectivism and individualism.
Even though British society has an individualistic orientation, British people
are still expected to take other people's needs and rights into account and may
face sanctions if we do not. Most cultures are highly complex and, in effect,
consist of numerous subcultures with very different values and aspirations.

It is easy to romanticize past ways of life, or ways of life remote from our
own, but values and patterns of behaviour can often be explained, at least in
part, by broad social, economic and political factors. In their book *Family and
Kinship in East London*, for example, Young and Willmott (1957) give an
account of the lives of working-class people in Bethnal Green. Their account
emphasizes the positive nature of social integration based on long-term resi-
dency, close family ties, and mutual trust, support and respect. Further analysis has revealed, however, that this way of life was maintained by poverty,
lack of choice, and lack of physical and social mobility. Feuds were common,
'outsiders' were not well accepted, and the community was maintained by the
oppression of women with men playing little part in community life other
than as wage-earners (Robb and Davies 1999).

Social, economic and political factors, such as poverty and gender inequality, are also influential in maintaining collective cultures in the majority
world. Foreman (1999b) points out that gender-based subordination is created and reinforced by religious and cultural beliefs and cultural practices
which assign women a lower status than men. Poverty, in terms of lack of
wealth, opportunity, power and access to services can also keep people
dependent upon their immediate community.

Communities with a collectivist orientation may be in a position to support those members who require it, for example frail, old people. In the absence of wealth or a welfare state, however, people are highly dependent on the productivity of each other. In many countries of the majority world the work of children is very important to the economic well-being and stability of the entire family unit and the notion of 'retirement' is unknown.

The juxtaposition of the concepts of 'independence' and 'individualism' can be very confusing. If independence is defined as self-sufficiency then it fits well with the doctrine of individualism. If, however, independence is defined as having control over one's life, then the involvement of other people may be vital to achieve that end. Collective provision, such as old people's homes, can, however, create dependency by restricting choice through limited resources or inappropriate services. Daunt (1991) points out that the tailoring of services to individual needs has nothing to do with individualism but is a demand that services which support the community, such as schools and hospitals, recognize diversity.

Another way of viewing independence is in terms of life transitions. As children and young people mature they make many transitions towards independence in terms of both self-sufficiency and control of their lives. The toddler who learns to run can use that skill to flout adult control and the child who learns to talk is able to argue her point of view. Children do not passively wait while adults decide what they can and cannot do but actively initiate, negotiate and demand new opportunities in their lives.

Two of the ways in which the transition from childhood to adulthood is achieved is through marriage or cohabitation, and employment and economic independence where it becomes possible to leave the parental home. In many countries of the majority world, however, children have adult responsibilities when they are very young through the necessity to work and the period termed 'adolescence' may barely be known. At times of war, or poor local employment prospects, young people may leave home and assume adult responsibilities earlier than would normally be the case. An extended education may hinder the transition to adulthood because of financial dependency on parents although it may enable young people to move away from home and have many new experiences.

Women in western society are no longer economically dependent on men so they do not have to wait for marriage before leaving the parental home as they did in the past. Many young people before the Second World War, however, went into service in their early teenage years as scullery maids, gardeners and kitchen assistants. This provided a partial transition to adulthood as, on the one hand, they were living away from home and earning their own wages, but, on the other hand, their meals and accommodation were provided. Their lives were, however, greatly restricted by the long hours they worked and the authoritarian regime imposed upon them although this may have afforded them some degree of protection.

It is clear that the meaning of independence and the ways in which it is manifested is determined by a wide range of cultural, historical, political, social and economic factors which are volatile and vary both within and among cultures.

Questions for discussion

1 How does the political doctrine of individualism relate to notions of independence?
2 How far do cultural, social and economic factors determine people's independence?
3 Is anyone really independent? Do you consider yourself to be an independent person? In what ways? In what ways are you dependent?

Disabled people and independence

Independence, in the narrow sense of physical self-reliance, is generally considered to be something disabled people desire above all else. Disabled people are admired when they strive for independence however inefficient, frustrating and stressful it may be. Being able to dress and wash oneself, walk, clean the house and make the bed are considered paramount however much time and effort are involved, whereas seeking help from others is rarely encouraged and may give rise to disapproval (French 1993a). Whole professions, for example physiotherapy and occupational therapy, have been developed to help disabled people achieve independence of this kind. Non-disabled people, in contrast, pay for cleaners, gardeners, mobility aids (in the form of cars and bicycles) and labour-saving devices without any sense of guilt or disapproval from others. Indeed the possession of such assets may serve as powerful status symbols.

Disabled people are, however, increasingly viewing independence in terms of self-determination and control and are rejecting the narrow, professional definition as oppressive and contra to their rights. This narrow definition of independence individualizes and depoliticizes disability and maintains a disabling physical and social environment (Oliver 1993). Ryan and Holman (1998: 19) state: 'Independence is not necessarily about what you can do for yourself, but rather what others can do for you, in ways that you want it done.'

Oliver (1993) contends that the dependency of disabled people is created by a variety of social, economic and political factors. Disabled people are excluded from the work place in large numbers which creates economic and social dependency. May (2000) points out that during the 1960s when jobs were plentiful far more people with learning difficulties were in open employment than they are today. Similarly during the Second World War, when many posts were vacant, large numbers of disabled people were given responsible work only to lose it when the war was over (Humphries and Gordon 1992).

Government policy, and failure to enforce policy, can also create dependency. In the Employment Act 1944 employers who employed 20 or more people were obliged to ensure that 3 per cent were disabled (the quota system) but this was never enforced. Health and community policy has created professional services that impose dependency on disabled people through institutionalization and inequality of power. Professionals act as gatekeepers to resources such as aids and equipment, and decide, in their role as 'experts', what disabled people can and cannot have. The language of professionals and social policy ('sufferers', 'carers', 'special needs', 'patients') reinforce the notion that disabled people are helpless and tragic. Davis (1993) has pointed out that professionals are dependent on disabled people for their careers, their status and their livelihoods and that many vested interests operate to maintain disabled people in their present situation.

It is often more difficult for disabled young people to make the transition from childhood to adulthood and to take control of their lives. As well as the barriers to finding work and being financially independent, their educational and social opportunities are more restricted because of hostile attitudes and an inaccessible environment. This, in turn, reduces the possibility of contact with their peers and provides less opportunity for friendships and intimate relationships to develop. Disabled young people, particularly those with learning difficulties, may be over controlled by their parents and carers and denied opportunities for experimentation and choice. People with learning difficulties may find it difficult to initiate change and parents and carers may be reluctant to do so because of upheaval, risk and a threat to existing sources of support.

Paradoxically many disabled children have been separated from their families and have been forced to be emotionally independent from a very young age. Lorraine Gradwell, who experienced early separation in a special residential school, talks about the effect of this:

> it left me with a high level of self-sufficiency or insularity . . . I think you develop reserves of self-sufficiency that you draw on in situations like that, especially in such a young child, and you haven't got your mum and dad around. The difficulty of not talking about things, you've no one watching over you . . . one of the long term effects is I am still quite self-sufficient, to the point that I probably appear stand offish to some people . . . it's a shame it had to develop.
>
> (quoted in French and Swain 2000: 24)

Although disabled people are usually regarded as the recipients of care, the notion of interdependency applies to them as much as anyone else. As well as providing work for professionals and others in the 'disability industry', disabled people give as much as they receive in their roles as parents, 'carers', employees, lovers, volunteers and friends. Institutions for disabled people, for example, could function only because of the work (largely unpaid) of the inmates, not only in cleaning, laundering and tending the garden, but also in assisting those who were more disabled than themselves. Andrews (2000), who has learning difficulties, explains:

We worked on other wards too, feeding, washing and dressing. We used to help the nurses . . . I used to make the beds, I did night duty too. I was knackered by the time I was finished. There was a tall lady who used to sit in this chair and she couldn't walk, not unless you walked behind her. So I had to put my hands out to stop her from falling backwards and I had to turn her round and put her on the toilet.

(Andrews with Rolph 2000: 36)

The government of Margaret Thatcher and the current Labour government have recognized the dependency-fostering culture of the welfare state and have sought to reduce the part it plays in people's lives. Various groups have been targeted including young unemployed people, unmarried mothers and disabled people. Oliver (1993) contends that although welfare services do force disabled people into dependency, reducing state intervention will serve only to condemn them to poverty and isolation. What is needed, he argues, are flexible services within a collectivist infrastructure which can be achieved only if disabled people have choice and control. It is not that disabled people want to be seen as independent but that the whole ideology of 'independence versus dependence' needs to be recognized as disabling and dismantled (Swain and French 1998).

Closely associated with the concept of independence is that of normality. Normality is a complex concept which engenders both fear and mistrust of difference while, at the same time, promoting individuality as a desirable commodity (Corbett 1991). People are expected to keep their idiosyncrasies and peculiarities from public display (Goffman 1976) and to present themselves as 'healthy, unlikely to cause trouble, motivated with an attractive image' (Fromm 1984: 146). The development of the concept of the norm or average in western culture can be traced to the early nineteenth century and is associated with the introduction and application of statistics (Davis 1997) and with evolutionary theory and a belief in progress (Baynton 2001).

The normal–abnormal construct is not neutral but is permeated with moral judgement and evaluation, with 'normality' being equated with virtuousness, and 'abnormality' with shame and scorn (Barnes et al. 1999). As Russell (1998) states:

When people do not run and jump, are blind or deaf, and do not exhibit able-bodied standards of physical or mental competence, nondisabled and some disabled people themselves perceive this as a 'less than' situation. These differences are interpreted as negatives, as 'not normal' and therefore, not desirable . . . The danger of the 'normal' construct is that it serves to make disabled people seem less than human.

(Russell 1998: 15)

Fawcett (2000) believes that the process of designating some people as 'abnormal' (and inferior) has the function of confirming the 'normality' (and superiority) of others. Talking of oralism, Baynton (1996: 55) states: 'The value of speech was for the oralists akin to the value of being human.

To be human was to speak. To sign was to step downwards in the scale of being.'

The normality–abnormality construct is an inherent feature of the medical model of disability where disability is perceived as an aberration which needs to be removed, corrected or hidden. This is translated into policy and practice in the 'disability' professions. Barnes et al. (1999) state:

> 'Able-bodiedness' becomes the benchmark against which physical and intellectual 'abnormality' are judged. This enabled the medical profession to focus its 'disciplinary gaze' on both acute and chronic conditions and as a consequence expand its sphere of influence to cover 'rehabilitation'. This 'medicalisation' of disability transformed the lives of disabled people. The medical interest was extended to include the selection of educational provision for disabled children, the assessment and allocation of work for disabled adults, the determination of eligibility for welfare payments, and the prescription of technical aids and equipment.
>
> (Barnes et al. 1999: 85–6)

Professionals may also believe that the ways in which disabled people function are inferior to those of non-disabled people. Tarver et al. (1993) state:

> Being in a wheelchair may give you mobility but it is a highly abnormal form of mobility with all kinds of disadvantages – practical and social. Communication through gesture or writing, or through a communication aid, is not normal human communication. It may be the only way to get your message across but it is still comparatively inefficient and open to misunderstanding.
>
> (Tarver et al. 1993: 7)

The pressure to be 'normal' is often at the expense of the disabled person's needs and rights. For example, if a person with a motor impairment who can walk short distances is denied a wheelchair, they may become isolated or unable to obtain certain types of education or employment. Mason (1992: 27) believes that 'almost any activity of daily living can take on the dimension of trying to make you less like yourself and more like the able-bodied' and Ryan and Thomas (1987) contend that the conventional and conformist lifestyles forced upon disabled people can be an exaggeration of normality. Sutherland (1981) talks at length of this, believing that,

> We are subjected to continual pressure to conform to a 'normal' image, this is one of the major reasons for the manufacture of elaborate prosthetic limbs and hands, which are often poor substitutes for the purely functional devices . . . which they replace.
>
> (Sutherland 1981: 75)

Making an impairment less visible (as is often the case with prostheses) can create social problems which are equally or more difficult to manage than when the impairment is exposed (Thomas 1999). As a disabled woman in Sutherland's (1981: 75) book explained, 'I'm happier with something that isn't a deception than with something that is.'

Many disabled people are well into adulthood before they manage to abandon, or at least challenge, these expectations of 'normality'. For most this is a gradual process which comes with the confidence of age, but for some it can be a sudden realization. A deaf woman in Campling's (1981: 36) book had such an experience, 'They were laughing and talking and didn't give a damn that the whole place knew they were deaf . . . My years of pretence seemed suddenly absurd. I had been making life "normal" and easy for everyone except myself.'

Morris believes that the assumption that disabled people want to be 'normal', rather than just as they are, is one of the most oppressive experiences to which they are subjected. She states that 'I do not want to have to try to emulate what a non-disabled woman looks like in order to assert positive things about myself. I want to be able to celebrate my difference, not hide from it' (Morris 1991: 184).

Abberley (1993: 111) believes that any abnormality which disabled people demonstrate results not from their impairments but 'from the failure of society to meet our "normal" needs as impaired people.'

Questions for discussion

1 What, if any, experiences have you had where your need to be independent, or your ability to pursue the lifestyle of your choice, has been impeded? How did you cope with this?
2 Why do disabled people disagree with the definitions of independence and normality which are applied to them?
3 Are professionals and disabled people interdependent?

Direct payments

One way in which disabled people have sought to take control of their lives is through the system of 'direct payment' whereby they receive a payment in lieu of social services. This, and independent living generally, has been achieved in the face of considerable opposition and scepticism by professionals. As Bracking (1993) states:

It is important to remember that the idea of independent living for disabled people as a right has evolved from within the disability rights movement – and not from within able-bodied society. To date, professionals' vested interests and public ignorance – or to be more accurate discrimination – have been major obstacles in our struggle for rights.

(Bracking 1993: 11)

The National Assistance Act 1948 made it illegal for local authorities in England and Wales to provide funding directly to disabled people, or for disabled people to employ their own personal assistants, although by the 1980s some local authorities were choosing to ignore this aspect of the law. Indirect payment, whereby money for personal assistance is administered to disabled people via a third party, was, however, legal and various trusts were set up for this purpose. Such schemes could also be administered by institutions such as voluntary organizations.

The first indirect payment scheme in Britain was developed in the 1960s by a small group of disabled people in Hampshire. They persuaded their local authority to rehouse them in the community and to use the money saved in doing so to pay for personal assistants. The payments were administered by the residential institution, Le Court Cheshire Home, where the disabled people had been living.

A major advance in independent living was the Independent Living Fund which was instigated in 1988. Funding was from central government and went directly to disabled people of working age to purchase personal and domestic services. Applications were means tested and assessment of need was carried out by social workers. The scheme was very popular and far outstripped estimated demand. By the time it was closed to new applicants in 1993, 22,000 disabled people were receiving payments.

Following years of intensive campaigning and research by the disabled people's movement, the Community Care (Direct Payments) Act 1996 was passed. It enables local authorities to make cash payments directly to disabled individuals who are 18 years or over in lieu of social services. The assessment of need does, however, remain with the local authority and the financial circumstances of the disabled person are taken into account when calculating the amount to be paid. Furthermore the direct payment can be used to buy only what the disabled person has been assessed as needing although some local authorities take a relaxed approach to this rule. Hasler et al. (1999: 54) quote a local authority manager as saying, 'Mowing the grass may not be in your assessment but once the resources have been allocated it should be up to you how you deploy them.'

Local authorities do, however, monitor how the money is spent and whether there is a surplus. Despite these shortcomings, Priestley (1999: 204) states: 'Direct payment legislation is an important policy development for the disabled people's movement. It challenges and undermines cultural associations between disability and dependence.'

The implementation of direct payments has been slow for all disabled people, but people with learning difficulties and people with mental health problems have been particularly disadvantaged. The legislation states that recipients of community care must consent to receiving direct payment. This can pose a problem for some people with learning difficulties although very often ways can be found to obtain consent by, for example, using alternative communication systems such as Makaton (a sign language), giving sufficient time, and ensuring that information is made as accessible as possible. The uptake of direct payments has also been slow among disabled people from ethnic minorities. Various barriers have been identified by Butt et al. (2000) which mirror problems of access to health and social services among ethnic minorities generally. This includes lack of accessible information, cultural insensitivity and racism.

The Direct Payments Act 1996 is a major breakthrough in the lives of disabled people that has come about through their own persistence, ingenuity and imagination. Many people find that the services they receive when controlling the resources themselves are superior to those provided by statutory services even though the cost is the same or less (Holman with Bewley 1999). Dawson (2000) found that disabled people value the greater flexibility that direct payment provides as well as the decrease in involvement with professionals and professional agencies. She quotes many people whose lives have been transformed by the policy, for example:

> With Social Service home care I feel that they came in, 'did me' and then went off and 'did' someone else, I was beholden to them. With Direct Payment I'm the boss and the employee has a different approach to me as I'm paying them rather than someone sending them to help a hopeless person.
>
> (quoted in Dawson 2000: 19)

Similarly Ryan and Holman (1998) talk of the transformed life of a man with learning difficulties:

> Peter has a hectic life now. He does the things that he wants to do. He really enjoys swimming, bowling and visiting museums. His itinerary is decided by Peter himself and his personal assistants explore new ideas with him. Peter indicates what he likes to do and when he wants to do it.
>
> (Ryan and Holman 1998: 22)

Priestley (1999) points out, however, that taken as an isolated policy, without social and environmental change, direct payment reinforces the idea that disability is an individual problem. He states that 'direct payments legislation is being played out within a needs-based system of distributive welfare rather than within a rights-based framework for inclusive citizenship' (Priestley 1999: 205).

Shakespeare (2000) also sees the contradiction between the individualism of direct payment and the collectivism of the disabled people's movement. He believes that the overall philosophy of individualism, as well as barrier removal and the need for personal assistance, needs to be addressed if the aspirations of disabled people are to be realized.

Questions for discussion

1 Why are so many disabled people in favour of direct payment? Are there any drawbacks?
2 Does direct payment conflict with the overall philosophy of the disabled people's movement?
3 What implications could direct payments have for professional practice with disabled people?

Debate activity

Debate the proposition: Independence concerns gaining control over your life rather than doing everything for yourself. The following quotations may provide you with a starting point:

> We know that we have to gain control over our lives even when we need help from others to function. Unless we do this, we can never make a real contribution to society because our own thoughts will never be expressed through our actions only those of other people, our 'carers' . . . Therefore we redefine 'independence' to mean having control over your life, not 'doing things without help'.
>
> (Mason 2000: 66)

> It was terrible . . . awful. I was independent before my accident and they [parents] were very good to me but they treated me as if I was about 6 years old . . . I wanted to do everything for myself and I thought if I stay here too long I'll just fall into the rut of letting them do everything and that will be the end really.
>
> (Oliver et al. 1988: 96)

Further reading

Davis, L.J. (1997) Constructing normalcy: the bell curve, the novel and the invention of the disabled body in the nineteenth century, in L.J. Davis (ed.) *The Disability Studies Reader*. London: Routledge.

French, S. (1993) What's so great about independence?, in J. Swain, V. Finkelstein, S. French and M. Oliver (eds) *Disabling Barriers – Enabling Environments*. London: Sage.

Oliver, M. (1993) Disability and dependency: a creation of industrial societies, in J. Swain, V. Finkelstein, S. French and M. Oliver (eds) *Disabling Barriers – Enabling Environments*. London: Sage.

Shakespeare, T. (2000) *Help: Imagining Welfare*. Birmingham: Venture Press.

8

Will you put your hand in your pocket?

Sweet or cold charity?

The topic for this chapter is charity and voluntary organizations. Charity touches all our lives inasmuch as it invokes a quality of interpersonal relationships. To be charitable is to 'give' and 'allow for' another person, ostensibly without personal gain. Here we concentrate on the institutional expression of such values through charity organizations and the meaning this has in people's lives, particularly those on the receiving end. There is perhaps no more fitting topic for a book about 'controversial issues' in that charity is perceived as both a positive and 'sweet' human value and a mechanism of social control and oppression. This is graphically portrayed in the novels of Charles Dickens, encapsulated in the notion of 'cold charity'. In the second section of the chapter we examine why disabled people have demanded rights not charity. The case study looks in some detail at an example of a newer charity. Connect is a charity which works with people with aphasia.

We begin, then, by defining charities in an organizational sense. Though there are many voluntary organizations that are not charities, and some charities that are not voluntary organizations, the terms are, for the most part, used interchangeably as they are in this chapter. In the provision of welfare, charities can be categorized as one of four response systems, the others being informal structures (most notably female family members), state provision and the private sector.

Rochester (1995) lists three criteria for qualifying for charitable status as an organization: to be independent of the state; to be controlled and managed by a committee or board of trustees who are volunteers (unpaid); and to exist solely to pursue charitable purposes of the relief of poverty, the advancement of religion, the advancement of education and other purposes beneficial to the community.

Voluntary organizations are highly diverse and fulfil a number of functions

(Kendall and Knapp 1995). The *service-providing function* involves the provision of a wide range of services direct to people. These include residential,
respite, domiciliary and day-care services; nursing homes, hospices, hospitals
and schools; legal services; and environmental services such as the preser-
vation of buildings. In his review of charities, Gerard (1983) found that three-
fifths of charities offer direct, client-centred services. He found, however, that
charities differed in their view of their relationship to state provision:

> About half see their activities as complementary to those facilities available
> from the state and half endeavour to offer a clear alternative to government
> provision based on different values and assumptions or a view-of-society
> and set of priorities which they do not expect government to share.
>
> (Gerard 1983: 150)

The *mutual aid* function is founded on the idea that there is a shared need
for security against risks and hardship and that if we all help each other we
will be helping ourselves (Beveridge 1948). Charity law, however, specifies
that a charity must benefit the public as a whole or a significant section of it
(unless set up to relieve poverty). Thus many self-help and mutual aid groups
are disqualified from charity status. The third function is termed *pressure
group*. This involves the collection and utilization of information in direct
action, campaigns and lobbying for change. Such groups include the Child
Poverty Action Group, Liberty and Oxfam. Again, however, overt political
action is not deemed charitable in law and organizations whose principal purpose is political change are excluded from the charitable sector (Rochester
1995). The fourth function is *individual advocacy* and involves presenting cases
on behalf of individuals to receive goods or services to which they should be
entitled. Finally there are the *resource* and *coordinating functions* that include
groups involved in liaison between voluntary bodies.

There have been sea-changes in charities and the voluntary sector over
their lengthy history. These have to be seen in the broader context of changes
in the economy, changing government policy and broad cultural changes
(Hanvey and Philpot 1996). As Mooney (1998) points out, however, it is also
important to consider how the past is relevant today. He shows how legacies
from Victorian philanthropy have endured and can be found, albeit transformed by social and historical context, in current debates. We shall mention
just four. First, social problems were, by and large, attributed to the inade-
quacy of individuals, as illustrated by the following quotation.

> There can be no doubt that the poverty of the working classes of England
> is due, not to their circumstances . . .; but to their improvident habits and
> thriftlessness. If they are ever to be more prosperous it must be through
> self-denial and forethought.
>
> (*Charity Organisation Review*, 1881, vol. 10, p. 50,
> quoted in Jones 1983: 76)

Second, there were believed to be different categories of poor people, particularly the 'deserving' and 'undeserving' poor. The former was to be supported

by voluntary charitable agencies, while the latter were to be provided relief in the workhouses. Third, it was widely believed that 'indiscriminate' charity would 'demoralize' and 'degrade' poor people. Finally, the dominant idea was that essentially social problems can be understood and overcome by trying to change individuals (Mooney 1998).

A more recent major time of change came immediately after the Second World War with the setting up of the welfare state, and the state assuming major responsibility for the welfare of its citizens. Though voluntary action was displaced most notably in the direct relief of poverty and the provision of hospitals, the charity sector was transformed rather than displaced. Some well-established charities, such as the National Society for the Prevention of Cruelty to Children, continued to make a substantial contribution, and a new series of organizations were established to fill the gaps and meet the perceived inadequacies of state welfare provision, such as SHELTER and the Child Poverty Action Group. More recently still (from the late 1970s) charities are increasingly being paid, by service purchasers, not just to fill the gaps in statutory provision, but to act as the agent of the state. Two key messages were propagated during the Conservative governments of 1979 to 1997: that collective solutions through an all-embracing welfare state have failed; and that problems are best addressed by a market-led system (Reading 1994). The growth of the market and contract culture was apparent throughout the Thatcherite era, and has continued relatively unabated by subsequent governments. So as voluntary income (from donations) has declined, the money from local and central governments has increased through contracts.

What then have been the implications for the voluntary sector experiencing this fundamental change of context? Though the diversity of the sector is such that it is difficult to generalize, a number of themes have emerged in the literature. Harris et al. (2001) summarize two widely recognized implications for the voluntary sector. First, voluntary organizations have increasingly taken responsibility for delivering 'mainstream' services that were previously provided by statutory organizations. There is a danger, then, that voluntary organizations will lose their distinctive character and simply respond to market opportunities offered by local and national state purchases rather than complementing or providing an alternative to state provision. Recent changes have tended to favour the larger organizations, and the survival of small-scale charities has increasingly been threatened, leading to less diversity. Becker (1997) suggests that many charities have found it difficult to cope with the increased demands on their services.

Second, the running and management of charities have become an increasingly complex and sophisticated task with increasing emphasis on accountability. Harris et al. (2001: 4) explain that 'commercial business practices became the preferred model for managing all organisations' and 'voluntary organisations were expected to demonstrate that they were "business-like" if they wanted to participate in the social policy market-place.' In this context, there is a danger that charity organizations become more self-serving, with resources being increasingly dedicated to the maintenance of the organization.

Another set of changes, sometimes contradictory to those mentioned above, come under the umbrella of 'user involvement', driven in part by the NHS and Community Care Act 1990, which make mandatory some user involvement in statutory services. Locke et al. (2001) found that most of the voluntary organizations they worked with had developed partnership or power-sharing between trustees or senior managers and users. This involved either 'a protected minority of places for users in formal decision-making bodies' or 'commitment to consultative procedures that feed into formal bodies' (Locke et al. 2001: 208). They argue that traditional charities may lose some of their share of the market as local authorities could turn to smaller community organizations that are closer to the users.

Questions for discussion

1 Charity is a set of social values as well as an organizational response to welfare needs. What meaning in terms of values does the notion of 'charity' hold for you?
2 Do you contribute to any charities (through donations of money, time and so on)? How and why?
3 What role do you feel charities and the voluntary sector should play in the provision of services, in relation to the statutory and private sectors?

Rights not charity

The dominance of charity provision in the lives of disabled people in Britain has been such that it is possible to talk of 'the charity model'. Historically this can be explained in terms of the role of charities in providing services and filling the gaps in mainstream state provision. Charities are also associated with the stereotyping of disabled people as dependent. Perhaps ironically, charity provided a bedrock against which disabled people responded in the establishment of the disabled people's movement. The Union of the Physically Impaired Against Segregation, for example, was founded by disabled people who left the segregated provision of Leonard Cheshire homes to live independently (Campbell and Oliver 1996). The role of charities in the growth of the disabled people's movement is evident, too, in the establishment of oppositional values characterized by one of the first slogans of the movement: RIGHTS NOT CHARITY. There is a further irony in that organizations of disabled people, including the British Council of Disabled People (BCODP) (see Chapter 14), have applied for charitable status. This was, however, a matter of pragmatism and political compromise to secure funding for the struggle for emancipation (Campbell and Oliver 1996). Notwithstanding any possible 'bounty' of charity, we shall concentrate here on the mass of continuing criticism emanating from disabled people against traditional charities.

Charities have been criticized on a number of fundamental grounds by disabled people (Drake 1996a). Traditional charities are led and controlled by non-disabled people. In his research, Drake (1996b) found that non-disabled people saw it as their natural role to run charities and they saw disabled people as the passive recipients of charity whose impairments prevented them from taking up leadership roles. Traditional charities are in the business of 'helping the helpless' and creating dependency (Charlton 1998). Furthermore, charities predominantly cater and provide for people with single impairments or medical conditions, for example the British Diabetic Association, the Multiple Sclerosis Society, the Royal National Institute for the Blind and so on. The 'charity model' is an individual model of disability which is closely associated with the medical model. Shakespeare (2000: 54) states that 'Charity is a way for individuals and society to avoid their obligation to remove social barriers and support needy members of the community.'

Yet traditional charities have held significant power in policy and practice decision making. They have both dominated negotiations with governments and taken up the mass of resources. At the time of writing RADAR (a government-sponsored disability organization controlled and run by non-disabled people) receives approximately ten times more state funding than BCODP. Oliver (1988: 10) writes: 'The time has come for them to get out of the way. Disabled people and other oppressed minority groups are now empowering themselves and this process could be far more effective without the dead hand of a hundred years of charity weighing them down.'

Charity advertisements provoke emotions of fear, pity and guilt, ostensibly to raise resources on behalf of disabled people. The images and language have built upon and promoted stereotypes of disabled people as dependent and tragic. Hevey (1992: 35) examines how charities market particular impairments and concludes that 'Charity advertising sells fear, while commercial advertising sells desire . . . charities promote a brand not to buy, but to buy your distance from.' These images are a highly significant component in the cultural construction of disability. Hevey (1992: 51) goes on to say that 'It represents the highest public validation of the isolation of disabled people. It presents a solution to the "problem" of disablement by a disguised blaming of the victim. It fails to find solutions because it itself is the problem.' And Keith (2001: 19) states that 'Whilst a lot of good may be done in the name of charity, it also creates distance and inequality between the giver and receiver; what disabled writer Nasa Begum has aptly called "the burden of gratitude".'

There have been recent moves by some charities to 'look at the ability, not the disability' (Barnes and Mercer 2001b). The Leonard Cheshire Foundation, for instance, had a national campaign focusing on the word 'en-abled' to accompany their move away from residential accommodation to other support services. Writing of such changes in advertising, Corbett and Ralph (1994) note the dilemmas that this has created:

The difficulty of changing image and focus within a conservative organisation; the tensions between the level of empowerment sought by those in the disability movement and that which charity proposes; the inadequate representation of real images in a desire to market attractive pictures.

(Corbett and Ralph 1994: 11)

Carr (2000) has presented a detailed critique of the Leonard Cheshire 'enable' campaign that echoes the concerns raised by Corbett and Ralph. She writes of 'the organisation which continues to appropriate our language as efficiently as it corrupts our image and commodifies our lives to ensure its thriving status as the leading charity provider for disabled people in the UK today' (Carr 2000: 29). She documents the repackaging of charity, to harness both the ideas of the disabled people's movement, such as 'Independent Living', and the cooperation of disabled people themselves, through 'user involvement initiatives'. Such strategies, she argues, are used to strengthen the charity model and the credentials of the charity in speaking on behalf of disabled people and rationalizing continued segregated provision. She concludes:

> The organisation is every bit as oppressive as it always has been and I'm sure no one involved in the disabled people's movement would doubt that but as we embark on our free our people campaigns, remember LC [Leonard Cheshire] is reaching for the sky at the moment . . . it's selling itself as a quality provider and has the wealth to capture untapped resources and markets.
>
> (Carr 2000: 35)

Russell (1998) has written in detail of the campaign by disabled activists against the Muscular Dystrophy Association (with telethon campaigns led by the comedian Jerry Lewis) in particular and charities in general. She writes: 'These two opposing images of disability, the charity model and the civil rights model, are on a collision course. While disabled people are intent on gaining dignity and equality . . . charities want to keep us back in Dickens's 19th century' (Russell 1998: 86).

Questions for discussion

1 Why are disabled people absent from powerful positions in traditional charities and why do agencies controlled by disabled people command fewer resources?
2 Why can the charity model and the civil rights model be said to be 'on a collision course'?
3 Why are the images of disabled people used in advertisements by traditional charities not acceptable to disabled people?

Connect: a new charity for people with aphasia

Connect is a charity which works with people with aphasia (language impairment) to provide appropriate services as they define them. It was launched in

August 2000 and moved into its present premises in south-east London in November of that year. The charity has its origins in the Department of Language and Communication Sciences at the City University in London where a group for people with aphasia was held. Sally Byng, who was interviewed for this case study, is the chief executive and research director of Connect. She spoke of the unease that she felt in her traditional role as a speech and language therapist:

> I found myself being presented with people with very complex life issues and I had absolutely no idea what to do about them . . . I always felt bothered that I was doing such a bad job.

Working as a researcher felt more comfortable but this was ultimately shattered by a growing understanding of disability from the perspective of disabled activists and academics:

> At the time I went to City, that was 1993, I knew nothing about the disability movement. It had never impinged on my professional consciousness until I picked up a copy of what was then *Disability, Handicap and Society*. From reading that I knew that, although my research met lots of scientific criteria, it was not satisfying from my point of view and was not morally and ethically sustainable. I was left with a profound sense of unease.

Connect was made possible by the receipt of a major grant from the Dunhill Medical Trust. The idea was to enable the work that had started at City University to spread throughout the UK. Sally described its philosophy:

> Firstly that it's possible to find new ways of living with aphasia. Aphasia comes as a big shock and disruption in people's lives but life goes on. People can find a new way and a new meaning to life . . . Our core philosophy is to share skills and share expertise. I don't like to label what we do. It's anti-tragic without minimizing what people are going through. We're working with people who are going through a period of major change . . . People find the meaning that they want. What we provide is a comfortable context so that people can do that personal exploration. The service we have here was very much driven by listening to people's stories which recast the whole experience of what it means to have aphasia.

Great thought went into the interior and exterior design of the Connect building in order to provide a welcoming, stimulating and accessible environment. In the first annual review of Connect it states:

> we decided to use colour to help people navigate the three floors, because some of the people who use our building have difficulty reading signs and reading numbers. These bright colours also make our building visually striking . . . We have seen how people's environments have even more impact on their well-being than we had suspected.

(Connect 2001: 4)

This is corroborated by Sally, who spoke of the impact the building has on people with aphasia:

> Some people have said that they often feel shut away and excluded – silent people, hidden . . . The whole building is very visible. It's making quite a loud statement.

There are no 'staff only' areas in the building which also gives a powerful message about the organization's culture.

A variety of services are provided at Connect with programmes and activities being negotiated with individual members. Most activities take place in groups where people can explore different forms of communication, have supported conversations and pursue leisure activities. A group of people with severe aphasia is, for example, developing new ways to communicate with people with aphasia in Australia and Israel. There is also a women's group, a self-advocacy group, a young person's group and groups for relatives and friends. A working group of people with aphasia is debating ways in which the recipients of the service can become more involved with Connect at every level of the organization. One of the aims of Connect is that people should feel comfortable with themselves and aware of the barriers that other people put in their way rather than seeing the problems they experience as *their* problems. It is stated in the first annual review that:

> Together people can engage in what it means to have aphasia and gain the confidence they need to find new ways of interacting with the world. They no longer feel excluded, instead they feel a sense of belonging . . . This inner confidence stays with people long after they leave the building.
>
> (Connect 2001: 12)

It is also thought important that family and friends have a good understanding of aphasia and can share their experiences and learn from each other. As Sally explained:

> Communication is a dynamic interaction between people so when we look at trying to support people to develop new ways of communicating we need to support the people around them.

As well as employing four speech and language therapists (one of whom is disabled), Connect employs a family support worker, two counsellors (one of whom has aphasia) and a group of volunteers. It also employs a fundraiser and administrative staff. Volunteers are currently being trained as 'conversation partners' who will visit people with aphasia in their homes and spend at least an hour each week in conversation with them. It is planned that this service will extend to assist people in accessing mainstream community services. Some people with aphasia who have used the services of Connect have become volunteers themselves.

Another major aspect of the work of Connect is teaching and research. Courses are run for people with aphasia, their relatives and friends, professionals and volunteers. These courses range from disability equality training to courses focusing on specific aspects of communication. Sally explained some of the difficulties of bringing their work to traditional health workers:

> We run training courses and that's a really big part of our work, and a growing part. We have very enthusiastic feedback. A lot of NHS staff are not happy with the service they deliver . . . a lot of people are feeling dissatisfied with what they can do so we have very receptive audiences. But it has to be a 'whole-systems' approach, you can't just have one player changing their behaviour . . . Some teams are trying to change but for me it's necessary to change the whole social relations of health care. What we say is that you need to work in a completely different way about completely different things . . . our problem is that what we do looks so unrecognizable to people. That is one of our challenges, to enable people to see what they can take out of it . . . Everything that we say is basic common sense. There's nothing clever about it at all. Sometimes I feel embarrassed about how basic it is.

Research projects undertaken at Connect always involve people with aphasia and are designed to be of direct relevance and benefit to them. For example, *The Aphasia Handbook* (Parr et al. 1999), which is designed for people with aphasia, was the end product of a research project sponsored by the Joseph Rowntree Foundation. It has won awards from both the British Medical Association and the National Information Forum for its clarity. A team of people with aphasia is currently evaluating web sites to see what is helpful to them so that the *Aphasia Handbook* can be made available on the Internet. Currently a research project entitled What Happens to People with Severe Aphasia? is being undertaken by researchers and people with aphasia both inside and outside Connect. A three-year evaluation of Connect has also been commissioned to ascertain the effectiveness of its services in the first year. The findings of research projects are disseminated, both nationally and internationally, through training programmes, conferences and writing.

A major aim of Connect is to influence mainstream services. Sally explained:

> Part of the point of setting up Connect was, not so that we could provide the best service for the few people who could reach us here, but in order to influence the way that services are provided through the NHS. That is really an important part of our identity as a voluntary sector organization. We're not an alternative service provider, we see ourselves as being there to support and influence the development of NHS services . . . We aim to set up a small number of these centres which we see as demonstration centres. They're test beds, experimenting with new ideas . . . We imagine that there will always be a role for something that acts in that way.

A new Connect project is up and running in the South West and a Connect centre is planned to open in Bristol by 2004. Rather than transposing the ideas and practices of the London centre, a great deal of consultation is taking place with people with aphasia who live in the Bristol area. The Bristol centre is likely to be different from the London centre because people with aphasia will be even more involved with the planning. Sally envisages the employment of a community development worker and that the work of the speech and language therapists will be even more grounded in a social context. She said:

It's about community reintegration . . . this is what bugged me all those years ago, the amount of contact time with people is a small drop in the ocean in relation to their whole lives – and their lives are just as complex as anybody else's. We need to find a sustainable way of supporting people.

Connect is new and is constantly evolving. Summing up its work in the first year, Sally commented:

It feels like people with aphasia are taking ownership of the place . . . I really believe that one of the fundamental things we've done is create the condition for them to do whatever they want to do . . . In the café it's just their place. They are the same people that used to come to City but their behaviour is so different here.

Questions for discussion

1 Is Connect an organization *of* or an organization *for* disabled people?
2 How far, if at all, are professional workers needed in an organization like Connect?
3 How far do you consider that Connect is underpinned by the social model of disability?

Debate activity

Debate the proposition: Traditional charities have been part of the problem rather than the solution for disabled people. The following quotations may provide you with a starting point:

one organisation has moved from being a traditional and, in some respects, paternalistic charity to having users as the majority of its governing body and its national and regional committees. It has become an organisation 'of' people with the condition it serves; users have a large share in 'owning' it, whereas once it belonged to a professional establishment.

(Locke et al. 2001: 208)

> The concept of charity, as defined by the courts, has an underlying social philosophy which has remained intact and has influenced the whole of our society's view of social welfare provision. Running consistent through the decisions is the idea of 'bounty'. 'Bounty' in the legal context means more than just liberty. Preserved within it, like a fly in amber, is a concept of social relations in which some people are active agents and others just passive recipients.
>
> (Williams 1989: 42)

Further reading

Charlton, J.I. (1998) *Nothing about Us without Us: Disability, Oppression and Empowerment*. Berkeley, CA: University of California Press.

Harris, M. and Rochester, C. (eds) (2001) *Voluntary Organisations and Social Policy in Britain: Perspectives on Change and Choice*. Basingstoke: Palgrave.

Hevey, D. (1992) *The Creatures that Time Forgot: Photography and Disability Imagery*. London: Routledge.

Lewis, G. (ed.) (1998) *Forming Nation, Framing Welfare*. London: Routledge.

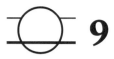 **9**

Whose body?

With Paula Greenwell

Theorizing the body

Since the early 1980s, issues to do with the body and appearance have increasingly been addressed by social scientists and we have moved into an era which 'can be characterised by its unique obsession with the visual display of identity' (Frost 2001: 37). A journey through any shopping centre will provide ample evidence of at least the economic importance of the body (commodification) – clothes to hang on it, jewellery, body piercers and tatooists to adorn it, soap and scent to perfume it, barbers to style it, beauticians to beautify it and make-up to paint it. It is evident too in the growth of keep-fit clubs and the number of joggers on our streets. The first section explores the wide, diverse and controversial topic for this chapter, 'the body'. The second section examines the significance of these issues in relation to disabled bodies, looking in particular at socially created impairment, sexual relations and medical technology and intervention. Finally Paula Greenwell has provided a case study as a wheelchair user with multiple sclerosis (MS).

As Hancock et al. (2000: 1) state, 'By the close of the twentieth century the body had become a key site of political, social, cultural and economic intervention in relation, for example, to medicine, disability, work, consumption, old age and ethics.' We look first at some key ideas that have emerged from contemporary debates about the body, concentrating particularly on theoretical perspectives. There are generally recognized to be two polarized perspectives on the body in the social sciences, though there are different positions within each. These are the naturalistic (including the biological and sociobiological) and the social (including the social constructionist) (Nettleton 1995). The contrast of the perspectives provides a basis for pin-pointing contemporary issues relating to the body.

The starting point for the naturalistic perspective addresses the body as a biological entity, irrespective of social and historical context, that determines what we are as individuals and our behaviour as social beings. A person's genetic make-up, hormonal activity and whole physical being can be drawn on in explaining desires and actions as a man or a woman. Within social psychology two types of explanations can be recognized. Causal explanations involve understanding the immediate predecessors of behaviours, thoughts or feelings. For instance, research suggests that the experience of emotion is determined by the interrelation of physiological factors (such as the release of hormones and heart rate), the social context and a person's understanding of the context (Toates 1996). Functional, or sociobiological, explanations start from the idea that our bodies are products of evolution. Natural selection is thought to favour those processes or mechanisms that best enhance the chances of the organism surviving to reproduce and passing on its genes. Human behaviour is seen as the culmination of a long evolutionary history. LeVay (1993) provides a succinct summary of naturalistic perspectives:

> People will ask of some trait – homosexuality, for example – 'Is it psychological or is it biological?' By that they generally mean 'Is it some nebulous state of mind resulting from upbringing and social interactions, or is it a matter of genes and brain chemistry?' But this is a false distinction, since even the most nebulous and socially determined states of mind are a matter of genes and brain chemistry too.
>
> (LeVay 1993: xii)

Critiques of naturalistic perspectives can focus on what is sometimes called essentialism. Essentialism is any way of thinking about human beings and social issues which suggests that behaviour can be attributed to 'essences' or fixed qualities. It can be argued that essentialist discourses legitimize inequality (Thompson 1998). Differences between people are seen as natural and therefore grounds for inequality. Supposedly natural sexual difference (the division into 'male' and 'female') is used to explain social differences. Inequalities between men and women are justified on the basis that 'men are stronger and more logical', 'women are better at caring' and so on. Saraga (1998) argues that essentialism implies both the permanence of a condition or identity and the homogeneity of people defined by this characteristic. She analyses a number of examples including sexual preference, ethnic minorities and disability. Of the last of these she writes, 'Disability is commonly seen as an essential, and hence permanent, characteristic of people, derived from physical/biological/psychological/cognitive traits' (Saraga 1998: 196).

There is now a growing body of literature that presents an alternative, social perspective. Though there are a number of different positions within this perspective, the central notion is that the body is socially constructed or created and how we think about our bodies depends on the social, cultural and historical context. Hancock et al. (2000) argue that the assumption that biology provides the dominant understanding of the body has collapsed and the meaning of the body has become a significant focus for linguistic, cultural and social analysis. Two important theoretical developments are the notions of 'body projects' and the 'somatic society'. Shilling (1993) sees the body as a project. He argues that the body might best be conceptualized as an unfinished biological and social phenomenon, which is transformed, within limits, as a result of its participation in society. Styles of walking, talking and gestures are perpetually in a state of 'unfinished business'. Furthermore, people try to alter or improve their appearance, size and shape in line with their particular desires. Body projects are, however, social at the same time as they are personal. Our perceptions and interpretations of the body are mediated through language and surrounding culture. Shilling (1993) argues that we live in an ever-changing world, ever more rapidly changing. Identity can no longer be derived from our traditional place within society, from class, family, gender or locality. The body, then, offers a site for personal control in a seemingly uncertain social context. He writes:

> Investing in the body provides people with a means of self expression and a way of potentially feeling good and increasing the control they have over their bodies. If one feels unable to exert control over the increasingly complex society, at least one can have some effect on the size, shape and appearance of one's body.
>
> (Shilling 1993: 7)

From this perspective, the body is not simply a personal project. In his often quoted and influential books, Turner (1996: 1) has proposed the notion of a 'somatic society' to denote a society within which 'major political and personal problems are both problematized in the body and expressed through it'. He has explored the social tasks in relation to the 'governance of the body' – reproduction, restraint, regulation and representation. In terms of reproduction, for instance, every society has to reproduce its members and developments in technology, such as in vitro fertilization and 'the pill', have considerably increased the control over reproduction (see Chapter 4).

He argues, then, that bodies are controlled, particularly by the institutions of law, religion and medicine. Turner builds on the concept of surveillance which has been significant within the literature. Foucault is particularly concerned with power relations and the body, and how control is maintained though inducing people to watch over their own behaviour. He says, 'Just a gaze. An inspecting gaze, a gaze which each individual under its weight will end by interiorizing to the point that he [*sic*] is his own overseer, each individual thus exercising this surveillance over, and against, himself' (Foucault 1980: 155).

Why has the body become such a significant subject for theory and analysis in the social sciences? There are a number of possible reasons. First, there has been a politicization of the body. An example of this is the way in which women have attempted to reclaim control over their own bodies from a male-dominated medical profession (Jacobus et al. 1990). Second, there are demographic factors. The proportion of old people in the population is increasing and the processes associated with ageing now form a substantial field of study.

It has been estimated that in Europe 70 per cent of disabled people are now over 60 years old. Third, there are many examples of deliberate cultural shaping of the human body in different societies and historical eras, such as the foot binding of women in traditional Chinese society, the cradle boards used to shape infants' heads among Kwakiutl Indians and the stays and corsets worn by nineteenth-century middle-class European and American women (Freund and McGuire 1995). More recently, however, the development of new technologies has opened up new possibilities for not only control of but also the shaping of the body. Shilling (1993) has pointed out that the more we know about our bodies and the more we are able to control, intervene and alter them, then the more uncertain we become as to what the body actually is. Turner (2001) writes:

> The transformation of medical technology has made possible the construction of the human body as a personal project through cosmetic surgery, organ transplants, and transsexual surgery. In addition, there is a whole panoply of dieting regimes, health farms, sports science, and nutritional science that are focused on the development of the aesthetic, thin body.
>
> (Turner 2001: 259)

Finally, there has been the rise of the consumer culture (Featherstone 1991). Identity has become a commodity, with the physical body providing the locus for consumption. You can buy the look, or purchase the lifestyle, though looks and lifestyles are, of course, not equally available to all. A consumer culture is essentially unequal. Images in advertising and the media sell 'the body'. Cultural representations of the body offer 'normative criteria' against which bodies are judged day-to-day. What is an attractive or even desirable body? We are all bombarded with almost unattainable media images of physical 'perfection', such as James Bond(s) and Bond's women. Gillespie (1998) associates this ideal of 'beauty' with the globalization of western media images:

> 'Mirror, mirror on the wall, who's the fairest of them all?' America's mirror screams back Blondie, Rapunzel, Cinderella, Marilyn Monroe, Christie Brinkley, Dianne Sawyer, Michelle Pfeiffer. Oh, yes, sometimes the look changes and those who are style arbiters decree brunettes, exotics or ethnics the latest 'in' look.
>
> (Gillespie 1998: 185)

It is in this social context that young women may be said to suffer from alienation from their bodies and experience self-hatred, which can become manifest in self-harm and eating disorders (Frost 2001). Kaw (1998: 168), in her study of Asian women undergoing cosmetic surgery, states that, 'Racial minorities may internalise a body image produced by the dominant culture's racial ideology and, because of it, begin to loathe, mutilate and revise parts of their body.'

Questions for discussion

1 What aspects of your lifestyle and identity as either a man or woman would you explain in terms of the biology of your body?
2 Thinking of your own physical appearance, were (are) you ever embarrassed about your body? If so, in what context and why? What would you change about your physical appearance and why?
3 Describe the physical characteristics of a 'good looking' man or woman in present-day western society. Describe a different set of physical characteristics of a 'good looking' man or woman either from a different historical period or from a different culture. How would you explain the differences between the two sets of characteristics?

Disabled body projects

To address issues generated by the question 'whose body?' immediately engages in controversy in the field of disability studies. This is essentially because questions about the body raise issues of impairment and can give credence to the medical model and notions of deficit and abnormality. Yet notions of 'body project' and 'body politics' are seen by some as challenging disability theory. There have been calls for the examination of impairment, like disability, as socially created and constructed and the possibilities are being sought for a social model of impairment (Paterson and Hughes 2000).

Most impairments are socially created and incidence is strongly related to demographic factors and structural inequalities. As French (1997) points out, in affluent countries, diseases now in evidence are chronic and associated with old age. These include heart disease, diabetes, respiratory disease, cancer, stroke, circulatory diseases, neurological diseases and arthritis. Visual and hearing impairments are also more common in old age. Furthermore, health and the incidence of impairment are unevenly spread across different sectors of society. Malnutrition, poverty and disease are very closely related. Impairments are also created by social phenomena such as war, traffic accidents, accidents at work and in the home, pollution and medical interventions. Meekosha (1998: 179) adds the effects of bodily interventions and conditions that particularly affect women: 'Early and unnecessary hysterectomies, the effects of drugs more readily administered to women, the connections between socially induced illnesses such as anorexia and later disabilities, and the disabling effects of cosmetic or medical interventions.'

The notion of the disabled body as a project has a long history, with the eugenics movement providing the philosophy and supposed 'scientific' justification for extreme measures of 'governance of the body', as illustrated by the following quotation:

The sociological conclusion is: Prevent the feeble-minded, drunkards, paupers, sex-offenders, and criminalistic from marrying their like or cousins or any person belonging to a neuropathic strain. Practically it might be well to segregate such persons during the reproductive period of one generation. Then the crop of defectives will be reduced to practically nothing.

(Castle et al. 1912: 286–7)

Eugenic practices involve measures to prevent the procreation of 'degenerates', including segregation and sterilization, and the termination of the lives of 'degenerates', including euthanasia. As Wolbring (2001) points out, today the main target for eugenic practices is the disabled body. The ideas of the eugenics movement persist today, for instance, in the perceived undesirability or inappropriateness of disabled people expressing themselves sexually. The disabled body is the site of oppression, abuse and prejudice. Sexuality is socially conferred and constructed rather than biologically defined and disabled people face social, political and economic barriers in their functioning and identity as sexual beings (Shakespeare et al. 1996; Lawrence and Swain 1997). Research conducted by Gillespie-Sells et al. (1998) suggested that most disabled women aspired to the establishment of sexual relationships, getting married and having children. They conclude:

> However, the study also showed that disabled women's opportunities to fulfil these aspirations are often not the same as those of their non-disabled contemporaries. Being continually regulated to lesser services, education, jobs and social opportunities all make it extremely difficult for them to develop and explore social contacts and relationships.
>
> (Gillespie-Sells et al. 1998: 119)

Disabled women are more likely than non-disabled women to be the victims of all forms of violence, especially sexual assault. There is a wide range of possible explanations. Dependence on care-givers, for instance, can render disabled women susceptible to abuse, unassertive in resistance and fearful of losing assistance (Cassidy et al. 1995). In the research by Gillespie-Sells et al. (1998), 29.28 per cent of the respondents said they had experienced sexual abuse by a member of their family, a further 24.31 per cent said they were victims of sexual abuse by someone other than a family member, and 48 per cent said they had suffered other forms of abuse. One Asian young person, interviewed by Middleton (1999: 10), responded to bullying in her own community by self-mutilation. She said, 'I did stupid things, like I rubbed my face with floor cleaner to make myself whiter. I cut my hair, I cut chunks off the front. There was one time I was so unhappy I got a knife and I cut myself.'

Another major set of issues concerns the subjugation of the disabled body to 'corrective' medical intervention, including cosmetic surgery, particularly associated with professional intervention to 'normalize' the disabled body. For many disabled people such interventions can be, at best, irrelevant and at worst abusive and dehumanizing. Nasa Begum (1994b), a Black disabled activist, for instance, writes of her experiences of regular sessions of physio-therapy during childhood. She said, 'I couldn't see the point of all these agonising exercises. I was never very good at accepting the fact that things I didn't like could be "good for me" and the physiotherapist managed to do a really good job of making me a conscientious objector for the rest of my life' (Begum 1994b: 48).

Four disabled people, interviewed by Johnson (1993), who had received physiotherapy had similar experiences to those of Begum and largely dismissed physiotherapy as having no importance in their lives. Also like Begum, a young person interviewed by Middleton (1999) rebelled:

> I hated physiotherapy, moving limbs about. I couldn't see an end to it. I was put in splints to straighten my legs, like callipers. I stood up all day: it was like a table on my back. I had to eat my dinner like that . . . I had no choice whatsoever. I was stood up all day from the age of ten to eleven. It was painful and demoralising, and when I was twelve I rebelled and refused to have the callipers on.
>
> (quoted in Middleton 1999: 18)

Meekosha (1998) writes of disabled women's experiences of cochlear implants, lengthening limbs, straightening body parts and facial surgery (for example on people with Down's syndrome). She states: 'These processes may be performed under the guise of indispensable medical treatment, but are in fact often designed to normalise the less than perfect body – to make it more attractive and pleasing, to fit dominant conceptions of attractiveness and desirability' (Meekosha 1998: 177).

Some young people Middleton (1999) interviewed had experienced 'corrective' surgery that was sometimes seen as a waste of time and sometimes conducted when the young people had other concerns and priorities. One stated: 'The arm was better when it was done but as time's gone on it's just gone back to how it was, because of the tissues there . . . Looking back if I knew then what I know now I would not have had the operation done. It messed up so many things at the time' (quoted in Middleton 1999: 21).

Questions for discussion

1 The statistics consistently suggest that disabled people are more likely to experience sexual abuse than non-disabled people. What explanations would you offer for the sexual abuse of disabled people?
2 List examples of positive images of disabled bodies in the media. What are the key characteristics of these positive images, and how do they differ from positive images of non-disabled people?
3 In what ways might experiences of medical intervention, particularly in childhood, effect disabled people's body-image?

'Was it fuck the MS'

The case study for this chapter takes the form of the story of one disabled woman. Paula is a disabled activist who is well known for her work with disabled people's organizations, particularly as chairperson of Disability Action North East (DANE). She agreed to be interviewed by John Swain, who is also a member of DANE. Paula had editorial control over the whole chapter. Her story is presented here in her own words, without analysis or interpretation, except through editing to the required word length. It is a story told in response to the topic for this chapter and, in general terms, addresses the question 'Whose Body?'

> For me there are so many aspects in this because when I was a young woman, I've always been very sociable but a bit of a loner. When I went through the usual puberty bit I emerged a swan from a duckling. I really got sick of men trying to chase me and women being jealous of me. The container I inhabited was a siren to the opposite sex, and I was saying I'm friendly, I'm warm and I'm funny and can we have a bit of that before sex please? Women didn't like me, because I was competition, and I didn't want any of that. I got sick of the fact that it was all or nothing. I felt at sea.
>
> When I was 22 I got MS and people said poor Paula she so loves to dance and I'm thinking well yes sure but there are lots of people that are perfectly fit and they've still got left feet. Been there, done that, got the tee-shirt. I'd done it. At the ripe old age of 48 I'd look a bit funny spinning on 4-inch heels. I felt sort of that I was inhabiting a body that didn't represent who I was. When I got MS obviously I was traumatised. My immediate instinct was oh no Jacqueline Du Pre and I can't even play the cello. For me MS simply meant increasing disability until death. So I thought, 'nice future'. A few years before I got MS people would say you should be a model and I was thinking what a fucking boring thing to do. For me that's what life is about, it's about new experiences. My body? Think about something more serious than that.
>
> The most important thing for me was discovery, creativity, learning new things, going to new places . . . for me it was 'see who I am' and that doesn't make any difference from a gorgeous teenager to a disabled middle-aged woman. It doesn't make any difference. I am who I am. And I will not be diminished because I should have been a beautiful but airhead person when I was a young woman. And now I am a disabled woman people think I have lost everything . . . and I have experienced so many things – sure it is a bugger being in pain, but it is part of who I am – I accept it. I am not angry about it. I have to get people to understand where I am coming from. Climbing stairs is not a challenge, changing the world is a challenge. People say 'oh you're a wheelchair-user this must mean you can't have sex', and I say 'why?' and they say 'you can't walk' and I say 'oh you walk while you are having sex?' I've got this wonderful irony which is a blessing. I don't understand why people accept status

quo. People say to me wouldn't you want to be normal and I say I wouldn't want to lower my standards. Who wants to be normal! You want to be like clones or something. I just had to do it a different way. It is part of who I am.

I know people with chronic illness they go to the gym three times a week. That would bore me shitless. The muscle in my head is the one I like to use. I got MS when I was 22. I was living with a guy at the time. I left him and I went abroad. Completely alone. I thought I had better cram this part of my life. I wouldn't swap my life for anybody's, not at all. My sex life improved when I said I was a disabled person. I came out as a disabled person. The biggest thing was coming off all the drugs. Coming off all the drugs I was multi-orgasmic whereas I had been struggling for years. I was thinking it must be the MS. Was it fuck the MS. It was the drugs. The anti-spasmodic drugs that I took.

Two of the best lovers I had were wheelchair-users. They were more imaginative. They were more sensitive and they were not performing. For me it is a very odd thing. I've been engaged six times. I've put up banns to be married in two countries. I love sex but I don't need it. I think that is personal to me. People think that I am desperate. It really pisses me off. I think it's something people make too much fuss about.

I am a communicator, first and foremost. A teacher, a lecturer, an actress, a writer, I am a communicator and that's what I need – and sex as well. I was sexually harassed rather than abused by my father. There are men that have said to me, 'you need me', and the answer is, 'I need you like I need a hole in the head'. This is the impression that they have of me as a disabled woman, that I need someone to support me physically and emotionally. What I want in a relationship is mutual respect and a lot of laughs.

The problem I have with doctors is that I upset them because it is the lack of need. I've seen a neurologist twice in two years and each time I've gone to him and I've said, 'anything new?' He gets really pissed off. I show him all the natural healthcare I take because I haven't taken drugs since 1986, that's why I'm in so much debt. What happened was when I got MS, you go to the doctor and you get a drug which deals with the symptom. I was taking these handfuls of drugs. A clinical ecologist said that people with MS are being slowly poisoned. I came off all the drugs and I felt tons better and I found that symptoms I had put down to MS were actually side-effects of the drugs I was taking, and I've been seeing natural health practitioners since 1986. It costs me a lot of money but at least I am coherent. This consultant I upset him because I take away his power and he doesn't like it. My own doctor he believes in natural health care so he is with me.

When I was taking the drugs I took them out of desperation with no discernible difference. They didn't help. So I have sorted all of it out. Years ago I used to lie awake all night with spasm, and cannabis stops that. We live in a world of superficiality, or comparison and we don't think beyond solids. We are so easily satisfied as a race.

I think that in some ways I have been out of communication with my body for some time, because it won't do as I fucking say, that's why. I think that the life that I have had has been extremely interesting. I am glad for who I am, and somebody else's body, it wouldn't be me.

When I first got MS, people used to say to me, 'I don't consider you to be a disabled person', and neither did I, and this goes to show what society knows of disabled people. They are largely ignorant. For me learning about the social model put everything in place. That's only bricks and mortar you can change that. So meeting other disabled people meant that I could use my voice to help the struggle. When people are demeaning to me or other disabled people personally most of the time I feel they are inadequate, I'm not.

Questions for discussion

1 How do Paula's experiences of her body differ from, and how are they similar to, your own?
2 Why do you think Paula has such a strong belief in alternative or complementary medicine?
3 In what ways might Paula have control over her 'disabled body project'? In what respects might Paula not have control over her own body, her embodied identity, and her experiences as a physical being?

Debate activity

Debate the proposition: The social model of disability, the disabled people's movement and disability studies have not considered the 'disabled body' and have, therefore, not addressed significant experiences of disabled people. The following quotations may provide you with a starting point:

> This can lead to the kind of absurd claims . . . that the disability movement has 'written the body out' . . . of all consideration. Quite how [he] comes to this conclusion when one of the central planks of the disability movement since Berkeley 1961 has been independent living is a mystery. Independent living is of course about nothing more or less than rescuing the body from the hands of medics, other professionals and welfare administrators.
>
> (Oliver 2001: 158)

> the weakness of disability studies' structuralist account is its failure to interrogate embodiment . . . The social model tells us little about the ways in which impairment is produced in the everyday world, how oppression and discrimination become embodied and become part of everyday reality.
>
> (Paterson and Hughes 1999: 608)

Further reading

Hancock, P., Hughes, B., Jagger, E. et al. (2000) *The Body, Culture and Society: An Introduction.* Buckingham: Open University Press.

Saraga, E. (ed.) (1998) *Embodying the Social: Constructions of Difference.* London: Routledge.

Shakespeare, T., Gillespie-Sells, K. and Davies, D. (1996) *The Sexual Politics of Disability: Untold Desires.* London: Cassell.

Turner, B.S. (1996) *The Body and Society,* 2nd edn. London: Sage.

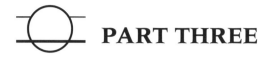 **PART THREE**

POLICY, PROVISION AND
PRACTICE

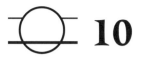 **10**

Policy: is inclusion better than integration?

With Tina Cook

Questions of inclusion

In the late 1990s policy debates in disability were dominated by notions of social inclusion (Oliver and Barnes 1998; Disability Rights Task Force 1999). We begin, as in other chapters, by exploring broader, general issues before turning to their particular manifestation for disabled people. Indeed, it can be argued that the first difference between the terms 'integration' and 'inclusion' is that the latter tends to have a broader remit. While integration has tended to be applied (though certainly not solely) to social policy in relation to disabled people, the notion of social inclusion tends to be applied to many groups, including old people and Black and ethnic minority communities. Integration has meaning in contrast to segregation. Disabled people have been subjected, and continue to be, to separate institutional provision in work, education, leisure and social provision generally. Inclusion, on the other hand, has meaning in contrast to notions of exclusion that have been applied generally to disadvantaged groups who lack personal, social, financial and political opportunities. In this first section of the chapter we examine what it means to be 'socially included' (and, of course, 'socially excluded'). We then turn to explore social inclusion in relation specifically to disabled people, focusing on paid employment and education. The chapter ends with an analysis of an ostensible move towards inclusive education in one local authority.

We begin by attempting to unravel social policy adhered to by the present (2002) British government. This is not as straightforward as it may sound as interpretations depend on the viewpoint of the observer (Roulstone 2000). In 1997 the British government set up the interdepartmental Social Exclusion Unit. It can be argued that social policy is being generated by notions of 'exclusion': 'A shorthand label for what can happen when individuals or areas suffer from a combination of linked problems such as unemployment, poor skills, low incomes, poor housing, high crime environments, bad health and family breakdown' (Social Exclusion Unit 1997: 1).

This idea of social exclusion has been widely adopted (Percy-Smith 2000) and has a long history with associated concepts of social disadvantage and deprivation. The main thrust in the government's response to social exclusion has been through paid employment, particularly New Deals to combat unemployment, but includes broader themes with, for instance, new funding programmes to support the regeneration of poor neighbourhoods.

In the first report on poverty and social exclusion, the government's strategy is summarized as follows: 'Our strategy is based in the principle that everybody has the right to participate in society, and the opportunity to achieve their full potential' (Department of Social Security 1999: Chapter 2, no. 27).

This quotation refers to universalism, participation and opportunity, that is widely accepted values in present-day western society. There are lots of questions, however. Who is socially excluded and why? Why has the notion of social inclusion come to prominence at this particular time and how does it relate to previous social policy?

Why does social policy begin with the notion of exclusion rather than inclusion? Beresford and Wilson (1998: 87) raise concerns that concentration on groups categorized as socially excluded may reinforce 'the lived realities of those who are included in its category'. Attention is taken away from the structures and relations within 'mainstream' society that generate social exclusion. Inclusion is conceived in terms of conformity (Burden and Hamm 2000). Social exclusion is individualized and pathologized.

In perhaps the most far-reaching radical critiques, social exclusion is seen as a natural constituent of late capitalist society. Levitas (1996) has written a widely quoted critique:

> The concept social exclusion, which was originally developed to describe the manifold consequences of poverty and inequality . . . is now contrasted not with inclusion but with integration, constructed as integration in the labour market . . . and treats social divisions which are endemic to capitalism as resulting from an abnormal breakdown in the social cohesion which should be maintained by the division of labour.
>
> (Levitas 1996: 5)

So social exclusion is a condition of society, rather than a condition of the individual. Some critiques argue that an inclusive society is not an achievable ideal in the context of globalization. Social exclusion is the natural consequence of deregulated global markets (Gray 2000).

From this viewpoint, then, the question in the title of this chapter 'Is inclusion better than integration?' is easily answered. Neither is better, as social inclusion is conceived as integration. Individuals are to be assimilated or integrated into existing mainstream society with no significant attempt to address the social and economic structures and processes that exclude people.

There is another understanding of social inclusion that has been increasingly developed within the literature, that is inclusion through widening and deepening of democratic practices and conceived in terms of full participative citizenship. Young (2000) states:

> The normative legitimacy of a democratic decision depends on the degree to which those affected by it have been included in the decision-making processes and have had the opportunity to influence the outcomes. Calls for inclusion arise from the experiences of exclusion – from basic political rights, from opportunities to participate, from the hegemonic terms of debate.
>
> (Young 2000: 5–6)

Beresford and Wilson have developed arguments for the inclusion of excluded people in debates about social policy. They suggest that 'debate about social exclusion can only be better informed if those directly affected are part of it' (Beresford and Wilson 1998: 91). Also, new participatory politics are grounded in the development of new social movements and the broad-based campaigns of Black people's, gay men's, lesbian and disabled people's movements. The inclusion of excluded people in social policy debates minimizes the risks of the pathologizing of social exclusion.

Questions for discussion

1 Do you think that social exclusion is a useful concept in social policy? Why, or why not?
2 How do you think the term 'social inclusion' compares and contrasts with the term 'equal opportunities'? How might they differ in generating social policy and strategies for social change?
3 Can you envisage a socially inclusive society? If yes, what would be the main features of such a society? If no, why do you think it is not possible to envisage such a society?

Social inclusion and disabled people

We turn next to explore social inclusion in relation specifically to disabled people, focusing on paid employment and education. Much of the emphasis on social inclusion of disabled people has revolved around their right to work and desire for paid employment, under such banners as 'from welfare to work'. As Oliver and Barnes (1998: 95) point out, disabled people are generally supportive of such a strategy, particularly as 'it is exclusion from the world of work which is the ultimate cause of the various other exclusions experienced by disabled people.'

The particular strategy of the New Deal and the Third Way taken by New Labour, however, has been subjected to significant criticisms (Hyde 2000; Roulstone 2000). Roulstone (2000: 429) states, 'it can be argued that policy thinking abjectly fails to acknowledge the weight of employment barriers that face disabled people' and current government policy leaves fundamental economic and social structures untouched. He writes of the rhetoric of the New Deal for disabled people which places the onus for social inclusion on disabled individuals, with employers facing 'little more than gentle exhortation to train and employ' (Roulstone 2000: 428). From their evaluation of a project which sought to create opportunities for paid and/or integrated employment for people with learning difficulties, Gosling and Cotterill (2000) state:

> The findings suggest that this goal can be undermined by many factors such as the isolation of social care services from employers and the disinclination of service organisations to include users, carers and staff in the development of new service approaches. Social welfare policies also mitigate against this aim, by failing to enable providers to translate the rhetoric of social inclusion into a reality.
>
> (Gosling and Cotterill 2000: 1001)

It is, however, the New Labour government's commitment to reduce the numbers of people claiming incapacity benefit, with a full-scale review of welfare benefits, that has generated the most anger among disabled people. In part it is based on 'an ideological separation of real and fictitious disabled people' and 'a clear attempt to separate out the work able (is this an unproblematic term?) from the "severely disabled" [sic]' (Roulstone 2000: 435). Britain, at the time of writing, pays over £6 billion in incapacity benefits to over 2 million claimants. In the latest round of proposals to cut this bill, all new incapacity benefit claimants will be required to attend regular interviews to check their continued entitlement to claim. Assessors will be able to rule that claimants are capable of work and should be transferred to jobseeker's allowance, a lower level benefit which can be withdrawn if it is found that the claimant is not genuinely seeking work (*Guardian, The* 2001). As Roulstone (2000) states:

> the 'New Deal' rhetoric of 'work for those who can' (regardless of the availability of work?) and 'support for those who cannot' could have disastrous consequences. People with perceived 'severe' impairments who are keen to work, may not receive the support they want in gaining work. People with hidden, but stigmatising conditions may risk being disabled by the additional label of poor outcomes in 'New Deal' terms.
>
> (Roulstone 2000: 441)

Rather than cost-cutting measures that increasingly emphasize the centrality of individual responsibilities, disabled people have called for a 'reappraisal of the very meaning of work' (Oliver and Barnes 1998: 96) and 'the general valorisation of non-working lives for those, including impaired people, who are unable to work' (Abberley 1999: 1). Questions of exclusion/inclusion are apparent within the education system as well as employment. The exclusion of disabled people from employment is mirrored by the exclusion of young disabled people from mainstream schools – and placement in special schools. Education policy and provision have highlighted the differences between 'integration' and 'inclusion'. The notion of inclusion has, centrally, shifted the debate from product to process. The focus for integration has been the numbers of young disabled people attending special schools (or mainstream schools). The focus for inclusion, in principle at least, is the processes of changing mainstream schools to be accessible to young disabled people, in terms of curriculum and teaching, organization, management, the physical environment, ethos and culture (Thomas et al. 1998).

Oliver (1996b) proposed that the term 'inclusion', as developed by disabled people from a social model perspective, should replace the term 'integration', as developed by politicians, policy makers and professionals. Table 1 attempts to summarize the main differences between the two.

Table 1 Integration versus inclusion

Integration	*Inclusion*
State: what matters is where young people receive education services	Process: what matters is the process of changing mainstream schools – curriculum, organisation, attitudes and so on – to reduce the difficulties in learning and participation experienced by pupils
Non-problematic: issues of integration are non-problematic and not questioned	Problematic: notions of inclusion raise fundamental questions about the provision of education in an unequal society and how this can be achieved
Education professionals acquire special skills: integration is solely a matter of extending the skills of professionals, largely through practice	Education professionals acquire commitment: inclusion begins with commitment to the development of fully accessible services
Acceptance and tolerance of young disabled people: integration is based on acceptance and tolerance of disability as personal tragedy and abnormality	Valuation and celebration of young disabled people: inclusion is based on the positive valuing and celebration of difference
Normality and equality of access: Integration is underpinned by dominant values of what is normal in terms of the person and the services	Recognition of difference: inclusion in services recognizes the diversity of need including race, gender and disability
Integration can be delivered: integration is professional led	Inclusion involves struggle: inclusion is partnership led, through negotiation

Source: after Oliver 1996b

> **Questions for discussion**
>
> 1 Should a social inclusion policy be led by the notion of 'from welfare to work'? Why, or why not?
> 2 Should opportunities for paid employment lead the social policy for disabled people of working age? Why, or why not?
> 3 How might the non-working lives of disabled people who are unable to work be valued?

Integration, inclusion and education policy

This is a case study of a local education authority (LEA) that we shall call Romantown, which has been reorganizing its special educational needs provision under a policy flag of 'inclusion'. The case study is based on research undertaken by Tina Cook and John Swain (Cook and Swain 2001; Swain and Cook 2001; Cook et al. 2001).

One aspect of Romantown's reorganization involved the closure of an all-age school (we shall call it Adamston) for pupils with physical disabilities, a school which first opened in the 1920s. The pupils from this school have been placed (September 1999) in a range of provision, particularly in mainstream schools with 'additionally resourced centres' and newly opened special schools for pupils with learning difficulties. (The reorganized system did not include a school for pupils with physical disabilities.) In this case study we explore and contrast the views of policy makers in Romantown with those of both some of the pupils who attended Adamston and their parents.

The Romantown reorganization was initiated and controlled by LEA policy makers, starting from the dissemination of their *Review of Provision for Pupils with Special Educational Needs* in 1995. This document set out the principles and policy that would remain unchanged throughout the 'consultation process'. This section of the case study is based on LEA documents and interviews with four LEA policy makers who were members of the Task Group responsible for planning the reorganization. We shall focus specifically on the notion of inclusion and its meaning in the reorganization of provision in Romantown. In the earlier documents relating to the reorganization the term integration was used rather than inclusion. In the LEA response to the Department for Education and Employment (DfEE 1997) Green Paper the term 'integration' seems to have been substituted by the term 'inclusion'. The Education Committee document states:

> [Romantown] LEA supports the principle that the majority of children with special educational needs should be educated within mainstream schools. The LEA considers that authorities should be required to submit plans for taking inclusion forward. Such plans have already been submitted by [Romantown] and are awaiting DfEE approval.

Inclusion became the preferred term in subsequent documents and in the interviews, and it is clear that the LEA regard the reorganization as a move towards inclusion.

In the following analysis of the Romantown policy we draw on a framework for critical analysis developed by Loxley and Thomas (1997) and using a thematic approach to identify key issues within the reorganization process.

Systemic dualism

A major theme for the Romantown policy makers was what Loxley and Thomas (1997) call systemic dualism, that is the continuation or discontinuation of dual systems of special and mainstream education. The main rationale for the reorganization of special needs provision in Romantown, as emphasized in public statements and documents disseminated by the LEA, was to enable a 'significant reduction in the level of segregation'. According to their own LEA *Review of Provision for Pupils with Special Educational Needs*, Romantown had one of the highest levels of segregation in the UK with over 2 per cent of pupils attending special schools. The maintenance and, indeed, enhancement of the special sector was also a recurring theme. This is apparent in the emphasis on 'the continuum of provision':

> the Task Group intends to progress the enhancement of the continuum of provision . . . both through the creation of a facility for a limited period of intensive support in a special school and by the additional resourcing of a number of mainstream schools. In some instances, additionally resourced provision will be in a form of a 'unit', that is a geographical area of the school.

Though the number of special schools in Romantown was to be significantly reduced, from ten to four, special schools remained a significant part of the provision in the reorganized system.

Two other forms of systemic dualism can be seen in Romantown's reorganized system that exist between and within mainstream schools. The first is between mainstream schools, that is schools with and schools without 'additionally resourced provision'. Two primary and one secondary school within the city of Romantown have designated 'centres', 'units' or 'additionally resourced provision' (the various terms used in the official documentation) for pupils with 'physical and medical conditions'. The second is the possibility of systemic dualism within mainstream schools, that is to say the differentiation in terms of management structures, resource allocation and the operation of separate provision within mainstream schools. The following quotation from the *Education Development Plan 1999–2002* certainly seems to indicate a degree of separation:

> The centres for the physically disabled population, in particular, have rooms equipped to cater for medical and nursing needs and have been adapted to provide full access. Planning has taken place in conjunction

with the Local Health Authority and City Health Trust and the centres will be jointly staffed with educationalists and therapists.

Resources

Issues around resourcing are a major theme in the documents and the interviews with policy makers. Indeed resourcing issues are generally given such a high priority it could be argued that 'policy decisions are shaped by an overriding concern with resource implications' (Loxley and Thomas 1997: 279). The position, repeatedly stated in Romantown, was that reorganization was a 'cost neutral' exercise, with the implication, sometimes specifically stated, that no extra resources would be allocated to meet special educational needs within the reorganized system.

Consumer centredness

Another key theme in Romantown policy is consumer centredness: the focus upon the needs of individual pupils, and the provision of services to meet their needs. The policy makers we interviewed emphasized the increase of choice available to parents through extending and improving the continuum of provision. Indeed, the policy makers consistently argued that the reorganized system allowed for an extended and improved continuum of provision. There would be a variety of provision for pupils with physical disabilities, according to their particular needs, namely in individual local schools, the additionally resourced provision in three mainstream schools or special schools for pupils with learning difficulties allowing placements to be individualized although not necessarily localized.

Democratization

A final theme we would pin-point is democratization, that is the involvement of parents and/or students in decision-making processes and valuing that involvement. Alongside the improvement in the continuum of provision, policy makers emphasized improved opportunities for parents to be involved in the choice of provision for their child.

All parents and family members interviewed were positive about the educational opportunities and wider support their child had received during their time at Adamston (a segregated school) yet almost all were also positive about the philosophy of children with special educational needs attending their local mainstream school, as illustrated by the following quotations from two mothers we interviewed.

Ideally I want my child to go to school with our next door neighbour.

Inclusion with so-called normal children, whatever a normal child is. He doesn't get it here.

However, the parents felt very strongly that the LEA had already made certain decisions about the shape of the reorganization and that their thoughts and ideas were not being valued. They felt they should have been brought into the LEA planning process right at the beginning so that their expertise as parents and carers could be utilized. They felt they had knowledge and information that could have helped the LEA to develop a greater understanding of the children's needs and their input could perhaps have resulted in alternatives to certain plans. One father succinctly expressed the frustration experienced by parents:

> Instead of sitting down and asking the parents how to go about it, they didn't. They said right we're closing Adamston, your kids will be in units, that's it and then they waited for everybody to shout and everybody to get angry rather than sit down with the parents and say, look this is what we're going to do, what do you think as a parent. But [the LEA officials] didn't, they stood there in their suits and said you will do this.

When interviewed about the reorganization many parents quickly pointed out that while there was an increase in the range of provision, it did not actually represent an extension of their personal choice for their child.

> This exercise of inclusion has made things worse . . . as far as I can see, because what's happened now is the other schools are going to say well actually we are not set up for that, these special resourced schools are meant to be taking you.

Some parents questioned the reorganization on the very basis of its conception. They questioned whether the intention of the LEA to be more inclusive would be borne out in reality, as exemplified by a quotation from the mother of a 10-year-old pupil:

> I don't know whether it will work as such, 'cos to me inclusion . . . to me meant they went to their local school with support. Not to say Grays [a mainstream school with an ARU (Additionally Resourced Unit)] because that to me becomes another special school because the majority of them will go there.

These parents were questioning the fundamental principles of the proposal in terms of its intention to develop inclusive provision for children with special educational needs. They pointed out that only a selected few pupils from Adamston were to be given access to a selected few mainstream schools. One mother expressed the commonly held view that 'inclusion' in Romantown meant fitting children to the system, rather than all schools adapting to educate all children.

> It will not work if the schools don't adapt for the special needs either. I cannot understand why they want them to go into mainstream schools when they're not adapting to all their needs.

The idea that pupils could or should be involved in policy making or even decisions about their placement in the reorganized education system did not arise for the pupils themselves or anyone else involved. They were completely excluded from the consultation process and did not attend their annual reviews at which decisions about their placement in the reorganized system were discussed. Only once did a pupil appear at her own annual review. She burst into the room asking, 'What are you saying about me?' The meeting immediately stopped and she was gently ejected. The decision at the meeting was that this 14-year-old should attend a mainstream school. No account has been taken of these disabled pupils' views in the planning of inclusive settings. No account has been taken of what these young people valued about their education, how their views might affect processes of change, or what they would look for, and need to feel included, in a so-called inclusive setting.

The disabled pupils at Adamston experienced the loss of their community, originally created by non-disabled people through a policy of segregation and then terminated by non-disabled people in the name of inclusion. Adamston was a small community that provided social, emotional and psychological security for these young people. It is not at all surprising that young people want to hold on to the community they are part of. The reorganization – closure of their school and placement in the new system – has been done to these young people. They (even more than their parents) have been powerless.

Questions for discussion

1 Do you think the changes in Romantown constitute an example of inclusive education policy being put into practice? If you do, or if you do not, on what basis do you make this judgement?
2 How might those most affected by the education policy decisions have been more involved in the decision-making process?
3 On the basis of developments in Romantown, is inclusion better than integration? Why, or why not?

Debate activity

Debate the proposition: All schools should provide education for all pupils irrespective of ability, ethnicity and impairment. The following quotations may provide you with a starting point:

> The history of the twentieth century for disabled people has been one of exclusion. The twenty-first century will see the struggle of disabled people for inclusion go from strength to strength. In such a struggle, special, segregated education has no role to play.
>
> (Oliver 1996b: 93–4)

A good education will address issues of inclusion and equality and participation, but there is a tension between education from the point of view of society, and education from the point of view of the individual; so I tend to argue that there are limits to inclusion that are not just practical but that there are ethical limits, which come about through the learner's expressing a choice, or parents expressing a preference which might not go along with what a larger group might think is in the interests of those people.

(Norwich 2000: 110–11)

Further reading

Disability Rights Task Force (1999) *From Exclusion to Inclusion: A Report of the Disability Rights Task Force on Civil Rights for Disabled People*. London: Department for Education and Employment.

Oliver, M. and Barnes, C. (1998) *Disabled People and Social Policy: From Exclusion to Inclusion*. London: Longman.

Percy-Smith, J. (ed.) (2000) *Policy Responses to Social Exclusion: Towards Inclusion?* Buckingham: Open University Press.

Thomas, G., Walker, D. and Webb, J. (1998) *The Making of the Inclusive School*. London: Routledge.

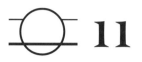 **11**

Provision: who needs special needs?

With Joan Adams

Who needs needs?

The notion of 'need' can seem unproblematic, particularly in relation to the fulfilment of what can be thought of as basic human needs, for food, for shelter, for security, for love and so on. The word 'special', too, can have positive connotations of exceptionality and distinction. Yet the concept of needs has played a key role in the unequal power relationship between professionals and disabled people, needs being defined and assessed by professionals in controlling the provision of services. The notion of special is also socially constructed, and largely given meaning for disabled people through segregation.

This chapter is about the use of language or discourse, that is ways of speaking, the words we use, the rules regulating what it is possible to say, who can say things, under what conditions and with what consequences. Hugman (1991) provides a good starting point for our discussion:

> Discourse is more than about language. Discourse is about the interplay between language and social relationships, in which some groups are able to achieve dominance for their interests in the way in which the world is defined and acted upon. Such groups include not only dominant economic classes, but also men within patriarchy, and white people within the racism of colonial and post-colonial societies, as well as professionals in relation to service users. Language is a central aspect of discourse through which power is reproduced and communicated.
>
> (Hugman 1991: 37)

We begin by exploring the concept of 'needs' and then turn to the notion of 'special needs' as it is applied to provision for disabled people. The case study analyses a particular example of the discourse of special needs in education.

One common concept of need is as a motivational or driving force. Perhaps the most well known theory of basic human needs as drives was first put forward by Maslow (1954). He suggested that there are five hierarchical levels of needs:

1 physiological needs (for food, sleep and so on)
2 safety needs
3 belongingness and love needs
4 esteem needs
5 the need for self-actualization.

The satisfaction of unmet needs lower within the hierarchy will, in theory, take precedence over higher needs. A child who lacks sleep and is chronically tired, for instance, will not be striving to fulfil needs for esteem through learning. While the hierarchy of needs might be generally useful, however, there are many exceptions, such as people in constant pain who still attend to 'higher' needs.

Doyal and Gough (1991; more recently summarized by Gough 1998) have developed the idea that human needs are common or universal in detail. The claim that physical health and personal autonomy are the most basic human needs is central to their theory of human need. These needs must be satisfied to some degree before people can effectively participate to achieve any other valued goals (Doyal and Gough 1991: 54). In this theory, citizenship rights follow from the concept of universal human needs as without adequate levels of need satisfaction a person would be unable to fulfil his or her duties as a citizen. Thus 'all people have a strong right to need satisfaction' (Gough 1998: 52). Standards of need satisfaction can be set and assessed. Such an audit, for these writers, is to be negotiated between the top-down knowledge of experts, professionals, researchers and so on and the bottom-up knowledge of ordinary people in their everyday lives (Gough 1998: 55–6).

This theory of need, from a different stance, however, feeds and rationalizes power relations that it purports to reject. Illich (1977: 22) succinctly characterizes an alternative viewpoint when he writes that, 'Needs, used as a noun, became the fodder on which professionals were fattened into dominance.' Professionals are dominant in power relations and structures through assessment of clients, defining their problems and needs, specifying solutions in terms of interventions to satisfy clients' needs, and evaluating the effectiveness of solutions. Needs are seen as residing in personal rather than structural deficiencies. In McKnight's (1981) analysis of professional services, he states:

> we see the professions developing internal logistics and public marketing systems that assure use of tools and techniques by assuming that the client doesn't understand what he [*sic*] needs. Therefore, if the client is to have the benefit of the professional remedy, he must also understand that the professional not only knows what he needs but also how the need is to be met.
>
> (McKnight 1981: 83)

Professional dominance can be seen in assessment procedures where, for example, the therapist's or nurse's observations may be viewed as objective whereas the patient's perceptions are viewed as subjective, and where pseudo-scientific language serves to mystify and confuse service users (Grieve 1988; French 1993b). Because of the specialization of the various professional groups, definitions of need tend to be narrow, their scope being dictated by specialized knowledge and interests (Ellis 1993). More recently, McKnight (1995: 29) has developed this analysis to turn the concept of needs on its head, and answers the question set by the title of this chapter, 'who needs needs?': 'Just as General Motors needs steel, a service economy *needs* "deficiency", "human problems" and "needs" if it is to grow . . . The economic need for need creates a demand for redefining conditions of deficiency.'

Questions for discussion

1 Is it possible to specify universal human needs (irrespective of historical, cultural, personal contexts)? If so what are they and how are they defined?
2 What would you say are your needs? Do they change over time and do they depend on context?
3 In what sense can professionals be said to need 'needs'?

What's so special?

What has the notion of needs meant for welfare provision for disabled people? First, when applied to disabled people, the notion of needs is often qualified by the term 'special'. While the term needs can be thought of as having universal application, 'special' is exclusive (in the sense of 'not ordinary') though again with positive connotations. It is synonymous with positive terms like: distinction, exceptional and extraordinary. Yet its application in relation to disabled people has been extensively criticized. Corbett (1996), in her account of 'the language of special needs' explains:

> Whilst it has the meaning within it to convey that which is positive, I rarely feel comfortable with the way it is generally applied. If 'special' is so positive, why is it not usurped by the patriarchy and widely employed to define power and status? . . . We reject being 'special' . . . When the term 'special' is applied to disabled people, it emphasises their relative powerlessness, rather than conferring them with honour and dignity.
>
> (Corbett 1996: 49)

Aids to mobility used by disabled people, such as callipers, are 'special aids', unlike non-disabled people's mobility aids, such as shoes. In terms of the provision of services, ostensibly to meet needs, 'special' has meant separate and segregated. Middleton (1997: 23) writes that, 'The invention and the persistence of the category in social policy hives off certain groups of people from mainstream assessment and provision, less for their own benefit than to maintain the quality of provision for those who are not special.'

The administrative separation of disabled people has dominated the service and welfare provision for disabled people, and enforced dependency. Priestley (1999), referring to the work of Barnes (1991), states:

Administrative segregation can be as powerful a form of surveillance and control as physical incarceration, if more insidious. In order to understand this point it is important to remember that British policy making continues to demonstrate an almost complete segregation of services for disabled people. Indeed, there are 'special' policies or statutes covering health, education, housing, transport, employment, social services, welfare benefits, sexuality, reproduction and civil rights.

(Priestley 1999: 50)

We turn next to look briefly at needs-led service provision first in community care and then education. Morris, who is a strong advocate of the social model of disability and the independent living movement, sees needs-led assessment as underpinning 'the development of services which will make a difference to people's lives' (Morris 1997: 44). She contrasts what she sees as a radical new way of service providers working in partnership with disabled clients with service-led approaches. The latter entails measuring the person against eligibility criteria to fit the person into a menu of services. She maintains that needs-led assessments are about: finding out what the client wants in their life; identifying the barriers; and creating opportunities to overcome the barriers experienced by the disabled person. For Morris (1997: 33), 'needs-led assessments are essentially based on a social model of disability.'

Other commentators are far more critical of needs-based provision. Oliver (1996b) recognizes that some benefits have been derived from the needs-led approach, including more access to relatively more services. Nevertheless he argues that there are serious problems. First, need is not easy to define. As mentioned above, Morris equates needs and wants, or at least derives the former from the latter. In the Doyal and Gough (1991) model, however, the two are clearly delineated. Second, Oliver (1996b: 70) states, 'above all else, assessment of need is an exercise in power', as argued above. A third problem with needs-led assessments is that they are undertaken in a context of fixed budgets, and the recent moves to charge disabled people for services. Priestley (1999) is unequivocal:

There is emerging evidence that the practice of community care assessment and management continues to produce packages of support which reflect traditional assumptions about the 'needs' of disabled people . . . By focusing the allocation of resources on personal care at the expense of social integration, the assessment process maintains a view of disability which characterise the needs of disabled people in terms of dependency and 'care' rather than citizenship and social integration.

(Priestley 1999: 105)

The needs discourse keeps the language of rights off the agenda.

Returning to the concept of 'special', nowhere in the literature of disability is the discourse of 'special' so dominant as in education. In the late 1970s, the

Warnock Report (1978) appeared to confirm dominance of the concept of special, particularly with its central focus on special educational needs, and the language of the report remains part of the language of policy as well as of daily discourse in mainstream as well as special schools. The spirit and espoused purpose of the report and the Education Act 1981 lay in the replacement of the categorization of young people in terms of impairment by the notion of a continuum of need. The central thrust was the reconceptualization of special education, then almost entirely equated with education provided in segregated special schools, to special provision for children identified as having special educational needs (SEN), many of whom were, and are, educated in mainstream schools.

In a sense, by extending understandings of special needs, the report and subsequent Act were successful, proliferating, if not spawning, an industry of special educational needs which remains. Warnock's desire to eliminate the categorization of young people by their impairments has not been successful. There has been some changing of terminology, from educationally subnormal (severe) (ESN(S)) to a superficially more humane severe learning difficulties (SLD), for instance, but three categories of pupils with learning difficulties are still used in educational provision: moderate learning difficulties (MLD), severe learning difficulties (SLD) and profound and multiple learning difficulties (PMLD), reflecting what Corbett (1996: 51) describes as a 'mania for categorising "special needs" into neat and distinctive sections.'

The DfEE (1997) Green Paper, which affirmed the Labour government's policy, retained the language of Warnock (1978) and the term 'special' recurred in a number of forms: special educational needs; special educational provision; specialists; special schools; special educational needs coordinators; specialist teaching; specialist support; and so on (Adams et al. 2000). Nor did the revised Code of Practice on the Identification and Assessment of Pupils with Special Educational Needs (DfEE 2000a) seek to address or change issues of language. In such official documentation it is therefore possible to identify a number of understandings of the term special at policy level, such as 'additional to', 'different from', 'greater difficulty in learning than' and 'a disability'.

In the two decades since the 1981 Act, specialness has continued to be institutionalized by the existence of segregated schools. There has been negligible change in the numbers of children attending special schools since 1990 (DfEE 2000b) and segregation continues to be promoted in government initiatives. Even the discourse around the changes necessary for integration (or the term increasingly used, inclusion) has largely been shaped by specialness. Thus, the Green Paper was able to refer to inclusion within mainstream schools, failing to recognize that within a truly inclusive education system there would be neither mainstream nor special schools.

In the development of more critical theories of the meaning of special in relation to education, a key text was Tomlinson (1982). She questioned the dominant humanistic explanations of special and traced the origins and growth of segregated education to particular vested interests, including those of medical, psychological and educational personnel, and political ruling groups. She also argued that the development of special education could be understood only in relation to development of the schooling system as a whole. She states that 'the 1944 Act allowed for a tripartite system of secondary schooling by "age, aptitude and ability". Selection by "ability" sanctioned selection by "disability"' (Tomlinson 1982: 50).

The wholly positive connotations of the term 'special' were and continue to be brought into question. A later paper, for instance, states that 'The special are likely to find more difficulty in collecting meaningful skills and competencies, having usually already acquired labels associated with "non-competence"' (Tomlinson and Colquhoun 1995: 199). More recently, analyses of the meaning of the term special have addressed the meaning of the term 'disability'. In particular, the social model of disability began to provide a foundation for a critique of existing essentialist theory and a basis for proposing radical change (Oliver 1984; Barton 1997). Riddell (1996) and Allan et al. (1998), among others, have argued that the official discourse of market-led educational policies has reinforced individualistic, rather than social, theoretical models.

Questions for discussion

1 Do you think that the concept of 'special' plays a role in the oppression of disabled people? If so, or if not, how and why?
2 Do you think that professionals need the concept of 'special'? Why?
3 How might needs-led assessments empower or disempower disabled people?

Teachers' conceptions of 'specialness'

This case study is based on research conducted by Adams (1998) in which she compared learning environments within one classroom for young people deemed to have moderate learning difficulties with another for young people deemed to have severe learning difficulties. One factor found to influence the learning environment was the teachers' own models of the 'specialness' of their pupils, with substantial differences between the two classrooms.

There were several perspectives in the way teachers talked about their pupils. Within the data evidence was first sought which related to the causes of the disability leading pupils to be given a statement of special educational needs. References to physiological symptoms were found only in the data from the SLD teacher who referred to pupils as having hemiplegia or a degenerative condition. There was little reference to pupils' cognitive level, and just one pupil was described as 'extremely slow'.

When the teachers of the MLD class talked about their pupils, they almost always described first their behaviour, and in negative terms:

Well, 8X presented a problem because of the outspoken comments and basically the cross-classroom conversations during lesson time.

If there's anything [science equipment] left out that you don't know about, you can find it being flung across the room.

They've had break time in the yard and you know you're going to spend the first ten, fifteen minutes of the lesson calming them down.

By contrast, they spoke positively about pupils' cognitive abilities:

The other day I gave Matthew a packet of sweets because he's so enthusiastic and he knows it. He's giving you all the answers all the time.

When you've got somebody like Scott and maybe even Luke at times who are quick on the uptake and know the answers straight away.

There's still Edward and Matthew who need to be watched as well. And when I say need to be watched in the sense, I mean they are two of the brightest ones in the group. I actually think Matthew's hyperactive, that's my theory about him.

In the school where the MLD class was located there were also pupils with SLD, taught in dedicated classes. Teachers spoke differently about these children considering, for example, that the SLD pupils more readily accepted differentiated work tasks. It seemed clear that there was variance in the way teachers perceived pupils with MLD and those with SLD.

There were differences too in the ways teachers interpreted the professional challenges that the two different groups of pupils brought. The MLD teachers, in seeking to understand and interpret their relationships with pupils, articulated a perception of distance, a social gulf between themselves and what they perceived as their middle-class values and those of the wider social world of the children they taught. Teachers felt that they were perceived by pupils as adversaries (one referred to herself as being seen as 'the enemy') and resented as figures of authority who made them do things they did not want to do.

At the same time there was a sense of discomfort with what they saw as over-familiarity exemplified by pupils commenting on teachers' dress or their families, or by suggestions that a teacher might participate in the social activities of day to day school life, by joining in a snowball fight. In contrast, the SLD teacher voiced empathy with pupils, identifying with their adolescent experiences, recalling that there had been times when she had acted, and reacted, as they did:

if I have to reprimand somebody, 'I remember doing that at school at your age' and the teacher would never have said that to me when I was at school. And somehow I say it because I think it helps them. I want them to know that I remember being like them.

She did not consider that their behaviours threatened her professional status as a teacher. When she identified problematic behaviours, she also had a solution that was within her control, 'he can be quite disruptive so I watch who I put him with.' This, ostensibly, positive and close relationship between teacher and pupil was attributed by the teacher to her understandings of pupils' impairments which required elements of personal physical care.

So, from the teachers' perspective, there are two individual models. There is an individual medical model that is applied in the education of children with severe learning difficulties. This model of special is conceived in contrast to non-impairment or non-disabled (disability being defined within the medical model). It seems that within this model, special is legitimized when applied to teachers themselves – special skills, techniques, curriculum. Special expertise is, supposedly, required for special children.

The second model, applied to children with moderate learning difficulties, could be termed the individual educational model. This model of special is conceived in contrast to perceived norms of capability, attainment but, primarily, behaviour. The model is more threatening to teachers as, by definition, these were children for whom, because of their behaviour, other teachers in mainstream schools had not been able to provide education. The very essence of special in this model, then, as applied to teachers' skills, techniques and expertise, is teaching ostensibly unteachable children. It is not surprising that the dominant approach to teaching in the MLD setting was didactic and controlling, particularly in enforcing the supposed norms of non-special education.

Questions for discussion

1 How can the discourse of 'special' be drawn upon to justify segregated educational provision?
2 In the light of these teachers' understandings of the term 'special', what are the implications for the development of inclusive provision?
3 In what ways might teachers' concepts of special needs pathologize disability?

Debate activity

Debate the proposition: The needs-led model of provision is inherently disempowering and segregationalist for disabled people. The following quotations may provide you with a starting point:

> Clear evidence of service development being influenced by a needs-led approach is an important incentive to, and reward for, the effort and thought which goes into needs-led assessment ... These changes are motivated by a shift away from fitting people into existing services, and instead finding out what it is that people want to do with their lives and using resources to make this possible.
>
> (Morris 1997: 43)

> the focus on 'needs' rather than 'human right' is in direct conflict with the concept of empowerment. The concept of need is an approach that runs through all the legislation and is one which promotes pathology, inadequacy and inability as the basis for determining who has what services.
>
> (Jones 1992: 38, quoted in Priestley 1999: 211)

Further reading

Barton, L. (ed.) (1996) *Disability and Society: Emerging Issues and Insights*. London: Longman.

Clough, P. and Barton, L. (eds) (1995) *Making Difficulties: Research and the Construction of Special Educational Needs*. London: Paul Chapman.

Corbett, J. (1996) *Bad-Mouthing: The Language of Special Needs*. London: Falmer.

Hugman, R. (1991) *Power in Caring Professions*. London: Macmillan.

12

Practice: are professionals parasites?

What is a professional?

This chapter concerns the role of professionals in the lives of disabled people. Although some disabled people have found the interventions of professionals and professional services helpful, others have been critical of the control professionals have over their lives and the restrictive nature of the services they provide. This situation has led disabled people to create their own innovative services which are based on their needs as they define them. This chapter begins with a broad discussion of professions and professionalism. It then examines the impact of professionals and professional services on the lives of disabled people. The chapter concludes with a case study of the Southampton Centre for Independent Living (SCIL) which is run and controlled by disabled people themselves.

The terms 'profession' and 'professional' are not easy to define and are used in a variety of ways. We may comment that the builder has done a 'professional' job, meaning that the job is done well, or that the shop assistant behaved 'professionally' when dealing with an awkward customer. When asked to name which occupations are professions, however, most people would not opt for builder or shop assistant but would probably choose doctor or lawyer though some may mention teacher, nurse or social worker. At its simplest level a profession can be defined as a particular type of occupation. The professions have been one of the biggest areas of occupational growth in advanced industrial society in recent years.

The 'trait' model provides one way of defining whether or not an occupation is a profession. This model defines professions in terms of distinct traits or characteristics (Abbott and Meerabeau 1998) although few professions encompass them all. These traits include:

- highly skilled work based upon theoretical knowledge
- the power to make autonomous decisions

- trustworthiness
- a service-oriented philosophy
- adherence to a professional code of conduct through a code of ethics
- a monopoly over a certain area of work usually through state legislation and state registration
- a professional body which selects, safeguards and controls its members by, for example, disciplinary action and the regulation of training.

Medicine, divinity and the law are frequently cited as 'pure' professions whereas occupations which have gone some way to acquiring these traits are referred to as semi-professions. The terms 'higher' and 'lower' professions are also used. Semi-professions include, nursing, social work, physiotherapy and teaching. Professionals are characterized by trust, respect and the belief that they work for the benefit of their clients. They are rewarded by autonomy, high status and, sometimes, high pay.

The specialist knowledge of professionals forms the foundation for developing philosophies, values and systems of work. Expert knowledge is thought to be essential if professionals are to be autonomous, self-regulating and trusted. Those occupations aspiring to become professions attempt to define their own body of knowledge and to separate it from 'lay' knowledge and the knowledge of other professions. In doing so they lengthen the period of training required, making it more specialized, and undertake research (Fulcher and Scott 1999). Many occupations, such as teaching, nursing and physiotherapy, have moved into the university sector since the mid-1980s where these aims can be pursued.

Hugman (1991) points out, however, that the trait model ignores the issue of power in the success of an occupation gaining professional status. The medical profession, for example, already had considerable power when negotiating its position with the state in the nineteenth century and when the National Health Service was introduced in 1948 (Ham 1999). With professions such as teaching and social work there is far less patronage by the state and more state control. The higher professions have been, and continue to be, dominated by men. A tiny number of women were admitted to medical school in the second half of the nineteenth century but it was not until after the Second World War that women were permitted to enter the prestigious all-male London medical schools. Restriction on the admission of women to medicine was outlawed by the Sex Discrimination Act 1975 and their number has been gradually increasing and now approximates 50 per cent.

Despite the high profile and respect that many professions and professionals have enjoyed, they have been challenged quite considerably by sociologists and feminists and more recently by the government who have attacked their exclusivity by introducing a 'market economy' into services such as health care and teaching (Nettleton 1998). Recent scandals, such as that of Dr Harold Shipman who was convicted in January 2000 of murdering 15 of his patients, has underlined the need for regulation and greater accountability on the part of professionals. Finlay (2000) writes:

the place of the profession in modern society has become a much explored area of discussion and research. Some scholars and commentators have been critical of professionals' power and how they maintain their advantage in society. Others suggest that professionals are losing their hold in the face of marketization, new regulations and consumer power.

(Finlay 2000: 74)

Those at the receiving end of professional services sometimes find themselves in opposition to professionals. Such people include gay men who may believe that they have been pathologized by receiving medical labels, and women who may feel that doctors are taking control of their bodies, in childbirth for example (Doyal 1998). Other critiques of professionals have come from ethnic minority groups who perceive them as ethnocentric, racist and lacking in cultural awareness and sensitivity (Ahmad and Atkin 1998). There is an unequal power relationship between professionals and their clients. Professionals have the power to assess and label people, to make moral evaluations about them and to define their problems. Their knowledge is regarded as reliable, valid and 'objective' while that of their clients is thought to be fanciful, dubious and 'subjective' (French and Swain 2001).

Professionals have been perceived, by their clients and sociologists alike, as controlling, distant, privileged, self-interested, domineering and the gatekeepers of scarce resources. Furthermore feminists have spoken about the patriarchal nature of the professions where high-ranking doctors and lawyers, for example, tend to be white, male and with 'social connections'. Davies (1998) states:

We need to recognise the cloak of professionalism for the outdated and male-tailored garment that it is. Nineteenth century ideas about what it was to be a responsible gentleman, to work hard to cultivate, not land but knowledge, and to apply it from a lofty and distant class position need serious amendment in the society of today.

(Davies 1998: 193)

The social status of professionals may thus depend more on existing power structures based upon gender, class and ethnicity, than on any claim to expert knowledge.

This alternative view of professions has been referred to as the 'power' model. It views the claims of professionals, for example expert knowledge and altruistic motives, as nothing more than rhetoric to justify occupational autonomy, privilege and self-interest. According to this model, skills are deliberately mystified (through jargon for example) to widen the gap between professionals and their clients and to increase the dependency of those who seek professional advice. Illich (1977) and McKnight (1995), for example, regard professions as disabling as they diminish people's ability to look after themselves.

Professionals have been accused of engaging in 'social closure' whereby they seek to maximize their rewards and status by restricting the opportunities of others, policing their own activities and monopolizing a particular social and economic niche (Abbott and Meerabeau 1998). Complementary practitioners are, for example, generally debarred from working within the NHS. If, however, they become sufficiently popular to pose a threat, traditional practitioners tend to take over their skills. Physiotherapists, for example, now practise manipulation and acupuncture within the NHS. Richman (1987: 227) contends that 'what is considered alternative medicine is the product of the powerful definers, who support establishment medicine.'

The Marxist view of professionals is that they are 'agents of social control', that is people who control and stabilize society on behalf of the state by individualizing social problems. This is achieved by focusing on and blaming the individual rather than dealing with social and environmental factors, like poor housing and lack of education, that promote inequalities in health and social problems such as crime and drug abuse. Thus a doctor may legitimize a few days off work for a stressed employee, or recommend a counsellor, rather than considering the environmental and organizational origins of the stress. In this way the status quo and the interests of powerful groups within society are maintained (French and Swain 2001).

As people have become more educated and have greater access to information and opinion via television, radio and the Internet, their deference toward professionals has diminished. Professionals live in ambiguous times being simultaneously revered and doubted, praised and scorned. It seems clear that their survival can no longer depend on professional status alone.

Questions for discussion

1 What makes contact with professionals, for example doctors or social workers, a positive or a negative experience?
2 Is it possible for individual professionals to change the system from within or do institutional structures make this impossible?
3 Do we need professionals?

Professional power: disabled people's experiences

The ideologies of the health, caring and teaching professions have had a considerable impact on the lives of many disabled people, not only in terms of policy, practice, and provision, but also on the way disabled people have been defined. Professionals have viewed disabled people as tragic, deficient and inferior and have sought to eliminate them (through abortion), remove them from society (through institutionalization), and to cure or approximate them to 'normal' through surgery, drugs and rehabilitation. Professionals have the power to assess disabled people, to define their needs, control the resources made available to them, specify solutions and evaluate outcomes. This, together with a disabling physical and social environment, has kept disabled people in a dependent position within society (Oliver 1993). Oliver and Sapey

(1999) contend that professionals stand between disabled people and the state as arbiters of need and, by doing so, maintain the status quo.

Some disabled people have found their relationship with health and caring professionals difficult and sometimes abusive. Michlene, a disabled woman interviewed by Sutherland (1981), states:

> My memory is basically of a whole series of experiences of being very coldly and formally mauled around. It's very alienating. It's as if you're a medical specimen . . . I was never told that I was nice to look at or nice to touch, there was never any feeling of being nice, just of being odd, peculiar. It's horrible. It's taken me years and years to get over it.
>
> (quoted in Sutherland 1981: 123)

Others have found difficulty, in the face of professional 'expertise', with being believed. A disabled woman interviewed by Begum (1996) said,

> If I don't get well they say it's psychological (hypochondria etc.). If it's psychological it's not really 'genuine' (apparently). If it's not real it doesn't need treatment. If it doesn't need treatment it's a sign I need to 'pull myself together'.
>
> (quoted in Begum 1996: 186)

Boazman (1999) had mixed experiences of professionals when she became aphasic following a stroke:

> Their responses towards me varied greatly, some showed great compassion, while others showed complete indifference. I had no way of communicating the fact that I was a bright, intelligent, whole human being. That is what hurt the most.
>
> (Boazman 1999: 18–19)

Disabled people have also found that health and caring professionals impinge on wider aspects of their lives. Professionals may be involved, for example, in decisions about employment, education, social benefits or whether or not extra time may be had in examinations. In that way the lives of disabled people can become increasingly 'medicalized'.

The treatment that disabled people have received at the hands of professionals cannot be dismissed as benign or misguided. Serious physical, psychological and sexual abuse have all occurred (Westcott and Cross 1996). Sam, who was interviewed by Corker (1996: 115), talked about the abuse he experienced at a school for deaf children: 'The more I was beaten, raped and abused . . . the more confused I became, wondering what I had done to deserve this. All this was made worse because I wasn't sure whether I could tell my father or how I could explain.' Mabel, a woman with learning difficulties, talks of psychological abuse:

> I never said anything in the hospital because there was no point. Nobody listened, so why speak? If you spoke they told you to shut up, so I stopped saying anything. I didn't talk, it was a protest really rather than anything else. I only said two words 'yes' and 'no', and mostly I said 'no'!
>
> (quoted in Brigham et al. 2000: 22)

Professional rhetoric is in terms of altruism and acting in the best interest of disabled clients. However, some disabled people have come to the conclusion that professionals are self-interested and are using them to secure a pleasant and lucrative lifestyle for themselves. In this way professionals are viewed as parasitic and dependent on disabled people. Davis (1993) states:

> It is a well established form of parasitism resting on bits of biblical dogma such as 'the poor always ye have with you' (John xii 8). The updated version of the old Poor Law, which sustains most of today's welfare professionals, depends for its continuity on such counsels of despair. It's become, let's face it, a nice little earner.
>
> (Davis 1993: 199)

Similarly, talking of researchers Oliver (1999: 184) writes: 'disability researchers are parasitic on disabled people, for without the host body (disabled people) there would be no disability researchers.' Teachers in special schools for disabled children have also been accused of vested interests and being more dependent on the children they teach than the children are on them. Tomlinson (1982) writes:

> The development of special education has been marked by a vast increase in the number of professionals who serve a clientele which they have vested interests in expanding. Literally, the more children thought to be in need of special education the more work for the professionals.
>
> (Tomlinson 1982: 83)

Professional practice has been strongly criticized by the disabled people's movement who view it as oppressive and abusive. It seems likely that the credibility of professionals working with disabled people will be discredited even further unless their practice changes radically.

Questions for discussion

1 Do professionals need disabled people more than disabled people need professionals?
2 How far are professionals losing their power in the light of critiques of their practice?
3 How, if at all, can professional practice change to become relevant and useful to disabled people?

An alternative service

Because of their dissatisfaction with professional practice and services, disabled people in many parts of the world have set up services of their own. Centres for Independent Living (CILs, sometimes called Centres of Integrated Living), for instance, are run and controlled by disabled people themselves.

Centres for Independent Living in Britain took their inspiration and impetus from CILs in the USA. The first CIL was opened in Berkeley, California in 1973 and there are now 300 similar centres throughout the USA (Charlton 1998). CILs have been established in most countries of the western world and in a few countries of the majority world, for example Brazil and Zimbabwe (Oliver and Barnes 1998).

Centers for Independent Living in the USA differ from those in Britain in three main ways. First, there is a stronger history of viewing social problems in terms of civil rights in the USA; second, there are fewer statutory services available to disabled people in the USA; and third, there is no large and established voluntary sector providing services for disabled people as there is in Britain (Oliver and Barnes 1998). In Britain CILs are linked, to some degree, with existing services and may rely on them for part of their funding.

Centres for Independent Living are run by disabled people for disabled people and provide many services including peer counselling, advocacy, maintenance of equipment, transport, training in independent living skills, housing and attendant services. Some provide extensive databases on issues relevant to disabled people, such as accessible holiday venues, and undertake disability equality training and research. They also lobby Members of Parliament and help other groups of disabled people to organize democratically. Their premises and information are accessible to disabled people with, for example, induction loops and information in Braille.

Equally as important as the many practical services CILs provide, is the challenge they pose to traditional services. Drake (1999: 190) states that CILs 'have proved a cogent and powerful alternative to the traditional gamut of projects like day centres and social clubs' and Oliver and Zarb (1997: 206) believe that CILs represent 'an explicit critique of prevailing social structures and the position of disabled people within them.' CILs also show that disabled people, rather than being passive victims, are capable of running their own affairs. As Finkelstein (1991) states:

> The fact that the centres and the services they provide have been devised and delivered by disabled people . . . presents a positive and rigorous public image contradicting the general depiction of disabled people as a burden on the state and an appropriate focus for the attention of charity.
>
> (Finkelstein 1991: 34)

Southampton Centre for Independent Living (SCIL) is a non-profit-making company limited by guarantee. The SCIL began in 1984 when a group of disabled people met to set it up. In the early days of the organization volunteers ran it but by 2000 it had 14 full and part-time employees and an annual income of over £200,000. The organization also has a large group of volunteers and an active management committee. Its main sources of income are from local authorities and the National Lottery Charities Board. The organization has no core funding and is, therefore, dependent on raising money from its own projects.

The aims of the organization are:

To provide a means by which disabled people may take control over their own lives, achieve full participation in all spheres of society, and effect change in how they are viewed and treated.

To provide encouragement, assistance, advice, support and facilities to individuals and groups wishing to live independently and to raise the expectations of disabled people, individually and collectively, and ensure their voice is heard.

(SCIL 2000: 1)

The work of the SCIL is based around 12 basic needs which have been identified by disabled people. These are for:

- an accessible environment
- aids and equipment
- personal assistance
- an adequate income
- advocacy and self-advocacy
- counselling
- accessible public transport
- accessible/adapted housing
- inclusive education and training opportunities
- equal opportunities for employment
- appropriate and accessible information
- appropriate and accessible healthcare.

The SCIL works in all of these areas, either directly or by collaborating with other organizations such as the Eastleigh Advocacy Service, which works with people with learning difficulties. In 2001 its funded projects were: to supply information and support to disabled people receiving direct payments; to provide disability equality training in a wide range of organizations; to assist disabled people in recruiting and employing their own personal assistants; to train disabled people to undertake consumer audit in local authority and other services; and to reach out to disabled people, particularly young people and those who are most disadvantaged, to help them take control of their lives. It also has an extensive database of information and produces information in accessible formats. The SCIL is a member of the British Council of Disabled People and actively campaigns in issues of concern to disabled people. The organization has been active in campaigning for comprehensive disability discrimination legislation and is currently involved in a campaign against disabled people being charged for essential community care services.

Centres for Independent Living have arisen from the personal and political struggles of disabled people and have engaged statutory authorities in a social model approach to services. They have blurred the distinction between users and providers (Priestley 1999). Barnes (1991: 223) states that CILs 'represent a unique attempt to achieve self-empowerment as well as being a form of direct action aimed at creating new solutions to problems defined by disabled people themselves.'

Finkelstein (2001) has argued that disabled people should strive to develop their own profession based on the new academic discipline of disability studies and the experience gained through organizations such as CILs. He names this the Profession Supplementary to the Community.

Questions for discussion

1 What is the underlying philosophy of Centres for Independent Living?
2 How do the services of Centres for Independent Living differ from traditional statutory services?
3 How far can professionals and disabled people work together to provide services for disabled people?

Debate activity

Debate the proposition: A wide range of professional interventions are necessary when providing services for disabled people. The following quotations may provide you with a starting point:

> We see our roles as providing 'consumer led' services and campaigning for the civil and human rights of disabled people. We believe that many services traditionally provided for disabled people have resulted in segregation, creating systems which actually increase passivity and dependence. We aim to work towards creating real opportunities for disabled people to live independently and to participate in the community. Our services are directed at empowering or enabling disabled people.
>
> (SCIL 2000: 1)

> Initial assessment . . . will be necessary to determine need with regard to medical matters, physical considerations, sensory impairments, psychological factors . . . social and family issues, personal finance, independence and day-to-day living matters. In addition, it will establish whether the client has aspiration or potential to retain or acquire paid employment. Particularly with regard to the latter, additional factors come into play, such as an assessment of the client's communication skills, numeracy skills, manual dexterity, educational and employment history and employment aspirations . . . The very broad spectrum of assessment dictates that the total process will, of necessity, be carried out by a team of multidisciplinary assessors working in an interdisciplinary manner under the leadership of a co-ordinator.
>
> (Etheridge and Mason 1994: 20–1, talking of the assessment of visually impaired young people for college)

Further reading

Davis, K. (1993) The crafting of good clients, in J. Swain, V. Finkelstein, S. French and M. Oliver (eds) *Disabling Barriers – Enabling Environments*. London: Sage.

French, S. and Swain, J. (2001) The relationship between disabled people and health and welfare professionals, in G.L. Albrecht, K.D. Seelman and M. Bury (eds) *Handbook of Disability Studies*. London: Sage.

McKnight, J. (1995) *The Careless Society: Community and its Counterfeits*. New York: Basic Books.

Priestley, M. (1999) *Disability Politics and Community Care*. London: Jessica Kingsley.

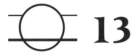 **13**

Policy, provision and practice: care or control?

What is 'care'?

This chapter examines the contested nature of the concept of 'care'. Although the word 'care' may be linked to warmth, closeness and love, it has also been associated with control, power and oppression. In the first section of this chapter the many meanings of 'care' and how these meanings are reflected in policy and practice will be explored. In the second section, the views and critiques of disabled people concerning 'care' will be examined. The chapter will conclude with a discussion of self-advocacy and will focus on MK SUN, which is a peer advocacy and campaigning group of mental health service users and survivors.

'Care' is a multifaceted concept with an ambiguous set of meanings (Hugman 1991). The everyday meaning of care, however, suggests concern and consideration for others. Caring for others and being cared for in return is important, indeed essential, for most of us. We feel happier and more fulfilled when others care about how we feel and what we achieve. Care can be expressed in many ways, by giving practical assistance, advice, emotional support, social support, physical intimacy and prayer. Caring is frequently reciprocal and may serve to strengthen relationships by increasing rewards, between say, close relatives or friends. It is not, however, always two-way, particularly as we may care about people we have never met, or those who have yet to be born. Even when reciprocity of care is not present, for example when caring for young children or a spouse with advanced Alzheimer's disease, experiences of providing and receiving care can still be valued. Caring is, then, ostensibly, a process of meeting people's needs, and concern for the welfare of others.

Despite these positive aspects, the notion of care carries negative meanings for many people and has been criticized by social scientists, feminists and those in receipt of care. Most carers are women and caring, as well as being devalued as a form of labour, is frequently seen as being a 'natural' component of the female character (Davies 1999). This idea has been strongly challenged by feminists. Brechin (2000) states:

> Caring, like mother love, risks being seen uncritically as warm, wonderful and quite unproblematic – and indeed, like mother love, is assumed to be richly rewarding and empowering for both parties . . . for some people warmth and support may be welcome, for others a more detached form of help and advice may be what is wanted, with 'care' seen as intrusive and inappropriate.
>
> (Brechin 2000: 141)

The cosy image of care as synonymous with love can serve to mask the control that operates in many relationships where one person is substantially dependent on another. Priestley (1999) contends that care within families frequently leads to possession and control, and Johnson (1998) makes the point that within social policy care is usually linked to control, supervision and protection. The social worker, for example, may, within an ideology of care, supervise people whose parenting skills are deemed to be inadequate, and young offenders may, at one and the same time, be subject to care, control, surveillance and protection. Talking of young people in residential care Ward (1997) states:

> For many of these young people, important decisions about their present and future life are likely to have been taken without their feeling properly involved and consulted . . . this general sense of powerlessness may add further to a sense which these young people have . . . of disaffection and alienation from adult society and its values.
>
> (Ward 1997: 238)

Physical, sexual and emotional abuse within contexts, which claim to be caring (for example families, children's homes and schools), is common with the most notorious cases appearing in the national newspapers.

McKnight (1995) analyses care in terms of the needs of professionals and the economy. He explains that as Britain's manufacturing industries have declined, the country has become increasingly dependent for its wealth on service provision which has resulted in categories of people being 'created' who are deemed to be in need of care. He states: 'More and more conditions of human beings are being converted into problems in order to provide jobs for people who are forced to derive their income by purporting to deliver a service' (McKnight 1995: 29). He cites the medicalization of bereavement, old age, 'hyperactivity' in children and childbirth as examples of this tendency. McKnight (1995: 39) goes on to say that the word care, 'masks the political interests of services . . . behind that mask is simply the servicer, his systems, techniques and technologies – a business in need of markets, an economy seeking new growth potential, professionals in need of an income'.

According to Adams et al. (1998) to be in receipt of care on a long-term basis equates with a very low social status. This, however, depends on the context in which the care is provided. As Shakespeare (2000) states:

if you describe a family who live in segregated accommodation, are looked after and have their meals cooked for them . . . have people to drive them around and are likely to be stared at wherever they go, it might be imagined you were talking about a very dependent type of person. Yet you would be describing the British Royal Family.

(Shakespeare 2000: 10)

'Care' services are generally stigmatized only if the person concerned is unable to pay for them or if they are heavily subsidized. When services are purchased they are usually thought of as 'support' or 'assistance' rather than 'care' (Brechin 1998). There is, for example, no shame or stigma attached to employing a cleaner, a gardener or a nanny or being pampered at a health club; indeed such assets and activities may serve as powerful status symbols. Similarly, having numerous servants was a sign of wealth and influence in the nineteenth and early twentieth centuries.

The meaning of care and who is deemed to require it varies over time and across cultures. Childhood, as conceived in western society today, for example, was constructed only in the late nineteenth century. This came about with compulsory education and legislation to control child labour. Until then, rather than being the recipients of care, working-class children were expected to work, obey and contribute to the economic welfare of their families (McCoy 1998). This situation still remains in many majority world countries today (Hewitt and Smyth 2000) where young children may also be enrolled in military service (Allen 2000).

In western society children have, over the course of the twentieth century, been viewed as needing more and more care and protection. The Children and Young Person's Act 1969, for example, stipulated that children who had offended were in need of care rather than punishment and the Children Act 1989 gave children greater rights under the law and more voice in what happened in them in, for example, residential care.

Such changes in philosophy within health and social care are reflected in language. During the eighteenth and early nineteenth centuries, for example, those in charge of mentally ill people were called 'keepers' rather than 'carers', which reflected their role in controlling and restricting the people in their charge. The term 'attendant' became popular in the second half of the nineteenth century and by the end of the century workers were referred to as nurses (Nolan 1993) which reflected the increasing medicalization of mental illness.

The concept of care has featured in legislation for many decades. Children, for example, were 'put in care' and people with mental health problems required 'after care'. In the NHS and Community Care Act 1990 the concept of care was substantially changed reflecting a market philosophy. Johnson (1998) explains that

> recent developments in state policy as a whole has reconceptualised care as a commodity for which people can be assessed and deemed eligible. It can be ordered, planned, managed, purchased, charged for, provided in the form of various services and marketed.
>
> (Johnson 1998: 152)

One way in which the concept of care has been broken down is the division between 'caring for' (labour) and 'caring about' (love) (Hugman 1991). 'Caring for' refers to the practical activities of caring (for example dressing, bathing, cooking and cleaning) whereas 'caring about' refers to the emotional aspects of caring (for example listening, comforting and explaining). Shakespeare (2000: ix) states that '"care" is a word which is value-laden, contested and confused, particularly in the way it combines an emotional component and a description of basic human services.' In reality 'caring for' and 'caring about' frequently occur together and the type of care which is appropriate depends on the person and the situation. 'Actions may speak louder than words' especially during times of acute illness or other crises. In addition many people express love and affection primarily by doing practical things for others.

The importance of negotiating with the person in need of support and giving that person control of their life is now recognized as a vital component of helping relationships. Talking of older people in residential care Peace (1998) states:

> For people who need the support of others to make real choices over how they live their lives, the staff need to be both enablers and doers, with the balance set through discussion. It is the imbalance of power of staff over residents which can tip what may be experienced as residential living into institutional care (or control?).
>
> (Peace 1998: 119)

People from ethnic minorities have been particularly neglected by health and social services as they have been expected to accept care which does not take their needs into account (Ahmad 2000).

The appropriateness of help and support will always be determined by the individual and their circumstances. Care can be both suitable and highly valued. Talking of their daughter's care in a hospice, for example, Zorza and Zorza (1993) state:

> Her happiness was clearly apparent. She had no guilt about being helpless and dependent on others. She had always loved to give, but she seemed at last to accept that she could now only receive . . . Her needs were fulfilled without question and without resentment.
>
> (Zorza and Zorza 1993: 230)

Questions for discussion

1 Think of a time when you needed care (either physical or emotional) from another person. What was your experience of this?
2 How did the other person's behaviour contribute to your feelings about receiving care?
3 Does care inevitably lead to control?

Do disabled people need 'care'?

Disabled people often feel stifled and oppressed by the care that they are given. Macfarlane (1996: 13) states: 'Many disabled people will define the care they have received as being oppressive, often of a custodial nature and provided in a controlled way.' Furthermore there is usually little if any control over who provides the care or the amount that is received (Oliver 1996b). Disabled people frequently find that others are taking responsibility for them, over-protecting them, controlling them, abusing them and thwarting their autonomy. Wood (1991) points out that disabled people have never asked for care and Morris (1998) states:

> In the context of the economic inequality which accompanies significant physical impairment in industrial societies . . . the need for personal assistance has been translated into a need for 'care' in the sense of a need to be looked after. Once personal assistance is seen as 'care' then the 'carer' whether a paid worker or an unpaid relative or friend, becomes the person in charge, the person in control.
>
> (Morris 1998: 167)

Walmsley (1996) found that if adults with learning difficulties lived with their parents the relationship tended to be one of dependency or ridden with conflict. If the disabled person moved away, however, the relationship was more likely to be supportive.

Receiving help which is excessively refined and 'professionalized' can also feel stifling and oppressive to some disabled people. Louise, a blind woman who we interviewed, explained how she felt as an employee of the Royal National Institute for the Blind (RNIB):

> People used to try out their new skills on you. I'd never heard of 'sighted guide skills' before I went to RNIB and people were all into trying it out on you, guiding you in the right way, and telling you the right thing – it all made me feel blind in a sense. Usually people do it fairly naturally or you tell them what to do. It made me feel very awkward and different and dependent.

Disabled people frequently prefer to train their own assistants rather than receiving professional 'care' (Morris 1993b).

Disabled people from ethnic minorities have pointed out that the care offered to them by health and social services is frequently inappropriate, inaccessible, culturally insensitive and racist (Ahmad 2000; Evans and Banton 2001). Vernon (1994) states that

> providers often assume that black families perceive it as their duty to care for their disabled relatives. It is also assumed by white professionals that black disabled people will be sufficiently taken care of by their extended family network . . . they may have to rely on their families to provide the care because of the inappropriateness of other forms of care to their needs.
>
> (Vernon 1994: 113)

In recent years, and particularly since the passing of the NHS and Community Care Act 1990 with its emphasis on 'care in the community', feminists have campaigned for the rights of carers. People in receipt of care have, however, been ignored in these arguments leading disabled feminists, such as Jenny Morris, to regard the debate as disablist. Feminist agendas have viewed disabled people as dependent and helpless and have therefore focused on 'the burden of care'. In so doing they have ignored the experiences of disabled people and colluded with prejudiced and discriminatory attitudes and behaviour (Morris 1998).

Disabled feminists and their allies have also taken issue with the assumption that disabled people are never carers themselves (Walmsley 1993; Morris 1998). Many disabled people who need some assistance are responsible for the care of children (Wates and Jade 1999) and other relatives (Walmsley 1993) or they work within the 'caring' professions (French 2001). Even if this is not the case, care is often reciprocal as Richardson (1989), talking about her adult son with Down's syndrome, explains:

> You are at war all the time . . . there is the emotional side of you which loves your child dearly and you don't want to part with him, there is the other side, common sense, which says now is the time . . . But there's a selfish side too, can I manage on my own? Am I going to be lonely . . . And financially, I had more for Martin than my pension now.
>
> (Richardson 1989: 9)

Disabled feminists have also been critical of the ways in which child carers have been portrayed without any regard for the disabled adults who need their assistance or the way in which society is constructed to create a situation where children are needed as carers (Keith and Morris 1995).

It is important never to be complacent about the care that disabled people receive. The history of residential care for disabled people is very bleak with numerous accounts of neglect and physical, emotional and sexual abuse. Stella recalled the time she spent in a residential school for visually impaired girls, during the 1960s:

> Even as nippers we were made to stand facing the wall for hours at a time. Quite regularly we would get the ruler across the legs really hard. There might be no sweets for weeks, or we were sent to bed without tea.

Quite often privileges like playtime were missed, instead we would have to stand in the corner very straight. We often got stopped from outings. I remember being stopped from a Christmas party, we stood from half past two until six o'clock facing the wall . . . We were marched out in front of the visitors and for tea we had cheese and watercress while all the other children had fancy cakes. The thing I did to deserve it was knocking the plants over in the playroom when I was running around. I just didn't see them but that wouldn't have been accepted, I was thought to be careless and naughty . . . It's vividly in my mind to this day.

(quoted in French 1996: 30)

Many other accounts of austerity and abuse of children and adults in residential care have been documented often by disabled people themselves. Potts and Fido (1991) have written a book based on interviews with people who spent many years in a 'mental deficiency' institution. Margaret (admitted in 1951) who was interviewed said:

If you were bursting to go somewhere and you wet yourself, you know like me, you got punished. Say you were in a wheelchair and you couldn't ask to tell them, you still got punished . . . couldn't go out, couldn't see your visitors . . . Shall I tell you something else, if you leave your food, you know what they used to do? If you didn't eat your dinner . . . leave it for your tea. And if you didn't eat it for your tea, you had it for your supper, and if you didn't eat it for your supper you had it for your next meal. It's true!

(quoted in Potts and Fido 1991: 59)

Mary Baker (1991) has written an account of the time she spent at the Halliwick School for Crippled Girls during the 1930s. She recalled her first day:

The nurse stripped me naked and cut my hair short. She couldn't have cut it any shorter if she tried. The sides were trimmed above my ears and I was given a fringe. The next part of my welcome was humiliating and degrading. My hair and my body was completely covered, sprinkled all over, with louse powder . . . I was being deloused but it made me feel dirty . . . The nurse told me there was nothing to cry about . . . Rules were rules and I had to be deloused.

(Baker 1991: 37)

Many other practices, which are undertaken in the name of 'care', have been identified as abusive by disabled people. These include medical practices (such as excessive physiotherapy), educational practices (such as preventing deaf children from using sign language) and attempts to 'normalize' disabled children by both their parents and professionals (see Chapters 6 and 12). Westcott and Cross (1996) have documented many recent reports of abuse against disabled children both at home and in institutions; Cross, who is herself disabled, has written a book for carers and parents which analyses abuse and aims to prevent it (Cross 1998). They both provide considerable evidence that the abuse of disabled children is more prevalent than the abuse of non-disabled children.

Since the development of the disabled people's movement, disabled people have developed a network of Centres for Independent Living which provide assistance on their terms (see Chapter 12) and have secured a system of 'direct payments' whereby they can purchase their own assistance rather than relying on what is offered by professionals (see Chapter 7).

Questions for discussion

1 Do disabled people ever need 'care'?
2 Do the critiques of 'care' by disabled people undermine the role of 'carers'?
3 How, if at all, can carers promote the interests of disabled people?

An alternative to 'care'

Self-advocacy means to speak out either individually or collectively and with or without support. It involves being assertive, standing up for one's rights, expressing one's needs and getting things done (McNally 1997). Self-advocacy groups work collectively to bring about change and to support and assist each member. They enable people to develop confidence and self-esteem and to learn valuable skills such as decision making (Gomm 1999). Self-advocacy has grown during the 1980s and 1990s as many marginalized groups, including people with learning difficulties and users and survivors of the mental health system, begin to speak out.

Advocacy, in contrast, involves a person speaking on behalf of another. In reality, however, advocacy and self-advocacy can be difficult to distinguish and may coexist. The goal of the advocate may, for example, be to enable the person represented to become a self-advocate (McNally 1997). Furthermore the advocate may be somebody who has gone through similar experiences. In this case the person is referred to as a peer advocate. Atkinson (1999: 5) states that the central thesis of advocacy and self-advocacy is that 'people's views matter and their voices should be heard.'

Collective self-advocacy has grown into a social movement which has enabled marginalized people, such as those with learning difficulties, to influence policy and practice. Self-advocacy has greatly expanded since the mid-1980s and has been assisted by legislation such as the Children Act 1989 and the NHS and Community Care Act 1990 which compel professionals to consult the users of their services. An example of a self-advocacy organization is Survivors Speak Out, which is a network of groups of mental health system survivors (Barnes and Bowl 2000). The organization was formed at a MIND conference in 1985 and the first conference of Survivors Speak Out, which took place in 1987, produced a Charter of Needs and Demands.

Although self-advocacy as a respected activity has only recently been recognized, it would be a mistake to imagine that marginalized people in the past were passive and silent. Talking of people labelled 'mad', Campbell (1996:

218) states that 'there has always been protest by mad persons at their negative designation in the eyes of society and at the systems societies have set up
to deal with them.' Early organizations such as the British Deaf Association
(founded in 1890) and the National League of the Blind (founded in 1898)
also stood up for their rights as disabled people. Ted Williams recalled taking
part in a march in the 1920s from Sheffield to London, organized by the
National League of the Blind, to protest against low wages and poor working
conditions:

> There was more or less a national uprising. The whole of England and the
> whole of Scotland decided to have a march to London . . . They arrived
> in Sheffield and all our workshops joined them and we marched down to
> London . . . we stood in Trafalgar Square and shouted for what improve-
> ments we wanted. We sent a deputation of shop stewards into parliament
> and I might add they got nowhere at all but it at least awakened people
> to our conditions.
>
> (quoted in Humphries and Gordon 1992: 117–18)

MK SUN, which stands for Milton Keynes Survivors and Users Network, is a
peer advocacy group where people who are experiencing or have experienced
mental distress help each other. There is also a campaigning element to the
organization where, for example, people are kept informed of changes in
legislation. Advocates and campaigners visit 'drop-in' centres and mental
health clubs to give information and offer assistance. I (SF) met the people at
MK SUN in 2000 when I was involved in making a video for an Open University course. The quotations below are taken from that video (The Open
University 2002). Karan Deighton, who is a peer advocate and the advocacy
coordinator, explained the work and philosophy of MK SUN:

> MK SUN offers a peer advocacy service, peers meaning that we're also
> users or survivors of the mental health system. We've actually been
> through the system so we know what we're talking about. The way that
> MK SUN Advocacy works is that we accept people's reality. If that's how
> they see life, that's where we go from. We don't judge them.

Part of the role of the peer advocates is to accompany people to meetings, for
example to see doctors or social workers, to help them get the most out of the
services on offer and to ensure that their voices are heard.

Paul Alsop explained his role as the campaign coordinator of MK SUN:

> At the drop-ins I can give the service users access to all the information
> . . . Only by raising the awareness of the individual can we hope to reach
> a point where mental health will be out in the open, not locked behind
> closed doors.

He also pointed out that, as well as being an advocacy and campaigning
organization, there is a strong social side to MK SUN:

> The 'drop-ins' are all friendly places. Everybody's in the same boat and
> working together and it's nice for people to have friends. It's like an

extended family that some of us lose when we become ill. When people become ill they lose an awful lot of their self-esteem. You go through the system and you're told what to do, when to get up, when to go to bed etc. MK SUN is a truly democratic organization.

Questions for discussion

1 Have you ever received help to speak up for yourself? How did you find the experience?
2 Why has self-advocacy become so prevalent in recent years?
3 Is self-advocacy a more appropriate form of assistance than that provided by statutory services?

Debate activity

Debate the proposition: Caring for disabled people inevitably leads to control. The following quotations may provide you with a starting point:

> I'd say we don't want to be cared for at all. I would say that we want to be facilitated, supported and empowered. Care to me has connotations of custody and lack of control and of looking after somebody who is sick and getting worse . . . I would say caring and care in the community is about control – maintaining us in a certain position – and it's about seeing disabled people as people with individual problems. It's not empowering at all.
>
> (Campbell quoted in Williams 1997: 94)

> They do everything for me, keep me clean . . . we cope between us . . . You couldn't ask any more. I've never lived in a hotel, I wouldn't know what it's like, but you couldn't get more attention by just ringing a bell.
>
> (Older disabled woman talking about living in a residential care home, in The Open University 1999)

Further reading

Cross, M. (1998) *Proud Child, Safer Child: A Handbook for Parents and Carers of Disabled Children*. London: The Women's Press.

Keith, L. and Morris, J. (1995) Easy targets: a disability rights perspective on the 'Children as Carers' debate, *Critical Social Policy*, 15(2): 36–57.

Macfarlane, A. (1996) Aspects of intervention: consultation, care, help and support, in G. Hales (ed.) *Beyond Disability: Towards an Enabling Society*. London: Sage.

Morris, M. (1998) Creating a space for absent voices: women's experience of receiving assistance with daily living activities, in M. Allott and R. Robb (eds) *Understanding Health and Social Care: An Introductory Reader*. London: Sage.

⊖ 14

Politics: where does change come from?

Social movements and social change

The topic for this chapter, 'Where does change come from?', is highly complex and fraught with challenging controversies. We look first at political change generated by new social movements and then look specifically at the disabled people's movement. As a case study of political change we analyse the British Disability Discrimination Act 1995.

Many social scientists accept that the period since the Second World War has been characterized by rapid and extensive social change – economic, cultural and political – both in Britain and globally. Some social scientists and commentators emphasize positive developments, such as the democratic and participatory possibilities offered by the Internet with open access to global communications, and the ostensible democratizing of the market with consumers free to choose with, for example, the expansion of television channels. On the other hand, more pessimistic analysts point to: the growing inequalities between rich and poor people both within and between nations; growing inequalities in access to global communication, including the Internet; the domination of the global economy by a few massive transnational organizations (including, for instance, Time Warner and Disney); and 'cultural imperialism' by the west and USA swamping minority cultures and reducing diversity (Held 2000).

Whether as an expression of positive globalization or resistance to negative globalization, a significant political change has been the development of new social movements, including feminist, civil rights, antiracist and community and welfare rights movements. Their role in mobilizing, organizing and exercising grassroots people power, and in 'citizenship expansion in the post-war period' (Turner 1993: 13), has changed the political agenda. As Fagan and Lee (1997: 144) state, 'women's equality, disarmament, decentralization, "race" equality, self-help – are now very much the stuff of modern political and social debate.' This is an arena of conflict between established top-down interests of those with economic and political power and the marginalized bottom-up challenges to the dominant order. Controversial issues proliferate, however, not least about how radical change can, if at all, take place.

Tarrow (1998: 4) defines social movements as 'collective challenges, based on common purposes and social solidarities, in sustained interaction with elites, opponents, and authorities.' Such 'collective challenges' have a long history and the question of what is 'new' about new social movements is itself contentious. Nevertheless, the development of new social movements has been associated with, among other factors, the breakdown of conventional work patterns, the growing gap between rich and poor people and overarching changes in the structure and nature of advanced industrial societies.

Giugni et al. (1999) documents some of the researched consequences of social movements, though recognizing that social change generated by social movements is not easily defined. They suggest that 'their consequences are often unintended and are not always related to their demands' (Giugni et al. 1999: xxi). The first set of outcomes are political, including changes in policy and their collective advantages for beneficiary groups, such as improved economic conditions or more equal opportunities for minority groups. The establishment of human and civil rights has been central to the new social movements of minorities marginalized by governmental structures and societal power structures and relations. In general terms, human rights can be thought of as the rights one has simply because one is a human being, and are held 'universally' by all human beings. Though there is a large area of overlap, civil rights can be seen as operating at a more specific and detailed level (Stone 2000). Civil rights (such as freedom of expression, of movement, and of religious practice) are sets of rights that either are, or ought to be, recognized by the public law of a political community and protected by the courts and law-enforcement agencies. Alston (1999) suggests that bills of rights have assumed particular importance in many countries in all parts of the world. He writes:

> One such example, the United Kingdom Human Rights Act of 1998, has attracted major attention within Western Europe, yet it is a drop in the bucket in global terms. In Central and Eastern Europe alone, there have been more than twenty-five new or revised constitutions drafted since the end of the Cold War.
>
> (Alston 1999: 1)

The Human Rights Act means that UK citizens can challenge breaches of the European Convention on Human Rights in the UK courts. Some of the main provisions include the right to life; to not be subjected to torture or to inhuman treatment; to liberty and security of the person; and to a fair and public hearing (Royal Association for Disability and Rehabilitation (RADAR) 2000; Stone 2000).

A second set of consequences is cultural. As McAdam (1994: 45–6) writes, 'social movements tend to become worlds unto themselves that are characterized by distinctive ideologies, collective identities, behavioural routines and material cultures.' Collective effort can take social change well beyond opposition to the political and economic establishment into the realms of culture and identity, such as the founding of feminist identity with the growth of the women's movement. Outlining the consequences of social movements, McAdam (1994: 51) includes the effect on the structure and curricular content of higher education in the United States, citing the establishment of African American, Native American, Hispanic and women's studies programmes. Social movements can also be seen as effective in bringing issues into public debate, such as sexual orientation and patriarchy in family relations.

There are some key issues generated by new social movements. First, questions have been raised about the predominant focus on the rights of citizenship. Some would argue that minority worldview of human rights is predominantly an individual rather than a community or collective approach. Legesse (1980) writes:

> In the liberal democracies of the western world the ultimate repository of rights is the human person. The individual is held in a virtually sacralized position. There is a perpetual, and in our view obsessive, concern with the dignity of the individual, his [*sic*] worth, personal autonomy and property . . . If Africans were the sole authors of the Universal Declaration of Human Rights, they might have ranked the rights of communities above those of individuals, and they might have used a cultural idiom fundamentally different from the language in which the ideas are now formulated.
>
> (Legesse 1980: 124, 129)

Turner (1993: 14) has also criticized notions of citizenship as repressive rather than progressive and as excluding outsiders and preserving the rights of insiders: 'under the bland moral shield of universalism, various types of particularity must be subordinated.' He cites the example of various aboriginal groups in, for instance, Australia and the United States and suggests that they are faced with two alternatives. They can opt for separate development within their own 'state', but this looks like a version of apartheid. Alternatively they can attempt to assimilate into existing patterns of citizenship, but this involves the inevitable destruction of aboriginal cultures.

Another set of questions concern the tactics of social movements. Is disruption or moderation, or a combination of both, more effective in realizing social change (Giugni et al. 1999)? The dangers of disruption include marginalization and denial of access to resources, while the danger of moderation is incorporation into the system and, thus, neutralization and emasculation.

Questions for discussion

1 What are your rights (human and civil)? Do you think you know your rights as a human being and a citizen? Why do you think that some people are more concerned about their human and civil rights than others?
2 What role do you think new social movements have played in political changes since the Second World War? Is social change generated by new social movements short or long term, significant or superficial? What evidence would you draw on in answering these questions?
3 What role has the feminist movement played in the changing identity of women and men in the post-war period, and what have been the main cultural changes emanating from the movement?

The disabled people's movement and social change

The disabled people's movement is thought by many disabled people to be a new social movement. Oliver (1990) points out that it is concerned with issues that cross national boundaries. Disabled Peoples' International (www.dpi.org) is an international umbrella group of organizations of disabled people formed in 1981. At the time of writing it represents over 160 national assemblies of disabled people, including the British Council of Disabled People, and is recognized by the United Nations as the representative voice of disabled people internationally. The stated aim of the DPI is 'to promote human rights of disabled people through full participation, equalisation of opportunities, and development' (Driedger 1989). According to Degener (1995), a German disabled lawyer, the role of organizations of disabled people is to increase pace of change in creating a legal framework to challenge the serious violations of the human rights of disabled people all over the world. There is ever growing demand to think about disability in a global context (Stone 1999b). Disability Awareness in Action (www.daa.org.uk), for instance, is an organization led by disabled people to increase networking among disabled people and their organizations worldwide. Speaking at a seminar in Sweden in 1995, Kalle Konkkola emphasized the DPI's mission as a human rights organization in the majority world:

> As chairperson I have felt that DPI's meaning is more important in the Southern Eastern and developing countries than in Western countries especially when we look at the level of commitment. Of course the organizations in Western Europe have commitment of working together but it appears as if the expectations on DPI are greater outside of Europe than in Europe.
>
> (quoted in Priestley 2001: 6)

Though it can be claimed that the disabled people's movement is global, the evidence suggests that there are different patterns of development in different parts of the world. Barnes and Mercer (1995) suggest:

> In the more industrialised North, campaigns have focused on the achievement of 'independent living' as well as 'full participation and equality' for disabled people. In comparison, economic conditions in the South have led disabled people to emphasize a different strategy in their struggle for emancipation – notably, the significance of community-based initiatives for economic participation and equality.
>
> (Barnes and Mercer 1995: 43)

Zames Fleischer and Zames (2001) have written an historical account of the development of the disabled people's movement in the USA. They suggest that a fundamental force in the evolving disability rights movement was the emergence of people with severe impairments from institutions and the independent living movement. Ed Roberts, the founder of the Berkeley Center for Independent Living (CIL) (see Chapter 12), states:

> we know what we wanted, and we set up CIL to provide the vision and resources to get people out and into the community. The Berkeley CIL was revolutionary as a model for advocacy-based organizations; no longer would we tolerate being spoken for.
>
> (quoted in Zames Fleischer and Zames 2001: 39)

The struggle for civil rights for disabled people in the USA followed the precedent set by the African Americans' rights movement. It was fought out, though less visibly, in the streets and the courts. It led to the landmark legislation in the field of disability, that is the Americans with Disabilities Act (ADA) which came into effect in 1990. Justin Dart, chair of the President's Committee on the Employment of People with Disabilities, stated:

> ADA is a landmark commandment of fundamental human morality. It will proclaim to America and the whole world that people with disabilities are fully human; that paternalistic, discriminatory, segregationist attitudes are no longer acceptable.
>
> (quoted in Cooper and Vernon 1996: 71)

A strong disabled people's movement has emerged in Britain in the face of the discriminatory barriers and oppression experienced by disabled people (Campbell and Oliver 1996). The movement consists of organizations *of* disabled people, that is organizations that are controlled by disabled people themselves. Organizations *of* disabled people are those where disabled people are in positions of control. A widely recognized key turning point for the disabled people's movement in Britain was the formation in 1974 of the Union of the Physically Impaired Against Segregation (French 2001). UPIAS was an organization established by disabled people themselves that fought to change the definition of disability from one of individual tragedy to one of social oppression.

The British Council of Organizations of Disabled People (BCODP, now called the British Council of Disabled People) was formed as an umbrella group for such organizations in 1981. A large group of member organizations comprise coalitions of disabled people and Centres for Independent Living which offer a range of services for disabled people and are controlled by disabled people themselves (Priestley 1999) (see Chapter 12). During the 1980s and 1990s BCODP continued to expand and, at the time of writing, represents 138 organizations. It articulates its demands through formal political channels, and lobbies and advises both central and local government. It also undertakes research (for example Barnes 1991), organizes demonstrations and campaigns of direct action, and promotes disability equality training.

The disabled people's movement continues to develop in a number of ways. Disability arts is a relatively recent, though well-established, branch of the disabled people's movement. A wide diversity of activities is encompassed within disability arts. There are a growing number of examples of the work of individual disabled artists expressing their experiences and communicating their thoughts and feelings, as disabled people, in many art forms. A central feature of disability arts, however, is collective experience. Disabled people are increasingly coming together to help each other express themselves in music, drama, forms of visual art and comedy. Through disability arts many disabled people have regular opportunities to share ideas and information with each other (see Chapter 6).

Turning to more controversial issues, questions have been raised as to the adequacy of civil rights in a fundamentally unequal society. Though stressing the importance of anti-discrimination legislation, Finkelstein and Stuart (1996) recognize that the possible gains are limited. More recently, Russell (1998) writes:

> Civil rights, although necessary to counter discrimination, may not be radical (get to the root) enough to change our predicament. Questions arise such as, how do economic rights factor into a globalized market that leaves greater insecurity in its wake and threatens to enlarge the 'surplus' population? What happens to universal concepts like full employment and a guaranteed income? Will civil rights solve the inequalities imposed by globalization?
>
> (Russell 1998: 127)

Scotch (2001: 390), too, points to 'the larger task of reorienting and redefining the disabling and institutionalized aspects of American culture and political economy'. In her far-reaching analysis, Russell (1998: 213) argues that the 'free market' is geared to the protection of the economically and politically powerful and has created a society that 'reduces personhood to a commodity, diminishing human dignity and eroding the human substance of the culture'. She calls for a fundamental shift beginning with 'democratic control': 'The people must have democratic control over all business: industry, banking, finance, land, commerce – the works – because without that, there can be no genuine democracy' (Russell 1998: 218).

The dangers of incorporation have also been recognized within the disabled people's movement. Barnes and Oliver (1995) put it as a dilemma:

> To get too close to the Government is to risk incorporation and end up carrying out their proposals rather than ours. To move too far away is to risk marginalization and eventual demise. To collaborate too eagerly with the organizations for disabled people risks having our agendas taken over by them, and having them represented both to us and to politicians as theirs. To remain aloof risks appearing unrealistic and/or unreasonable, and denies possible access to much needed resources.
>
> (Barnes and Oliver 1995: 115)

This reflects the division between 'reformists', who believe the system can be changed from within, and the 'radicals', who maintain that the struggle for change is compromised as organizations and individual activists are co-opted into dominant power structures (Barnes and Mercer 2001a). In his editorial to an edition of the activist journal, *Coalition*, entitled 'Where have all the activists gone', Lumb (2000) writes of the moderation line increasingly taken by the BCODP:

> One consequence of this was that much of the language of an oppressed group was gradually replaced by a language of 'reasonableness' adopted, no doubt, because of its acceptability to decision makers and, in the longer term, to secure and maintain a 'seat at the table'.
>
> (Lumb 2000: 4)

Finkelstein, who argued in 1996 that the movement had lost its vision for change, has more recently put these developments in a wider context:

> Emancipation movements are usually started by people on the political left but as the newborn movement manages to fumble its way through the first muddy barriers, not without casualties, individuals to the centre and the right of the political spectrum all too often 'discover' the movement's message and claim it for their own.
>
> (Finkelstein 2001: 13)

Yet many disabled people hope for change, and hope,

> is based on a strong conviction that current conditions and relations are not natural, proper or eternal. They can be changed. Hope therefore, can mobilise, galvanise and inspire. It arises from within a social context characterised by unacceptable inequalities and discrimination.
>
> (Barton 2001: 4)

Oliver (2001: 159) puts it succinctly: 'I remain optimistic and expect the next epoch to be much more inclusive than the previous one.'

Questions for discussion

1 What does it mean to say 'disability is a civil rights issue'? Why have disabled people struggled for civil rights legislation?
2 What were the main factors in the social and historical context precipitating the development of the disabled people's movement? What might have been the main barriers to the development of the movement?
3 How effective do you think the disabled people's movement has been in generating long-term significant social change for disabled people in the establishment of full participative citizenship?

The British Disability Discrimination Act 1995

With the growing influence of the disabled people's movement and the persistent demand for civil rights from disabled people during the 1980s and 1990s, the social model of disability has gradually become more influential and led in 1995 to the passing of the first Disability Discrimination Act in Britain. The Act, at least in principle, establishes new rights for disabled people in the area of employment, the provision of goods and services, and buying and renting land and property (Doyle 2000). Employers are expected to take 'reasonable measures' to ensure that they are not discriminating against disabled people. Although the legislation is weak, with numerous exemptions, Gooding (1996) describes its introduction as 'a fundamental shift'.

The Act provides the most comprehensive anti-discrimination legislation in Britain to date but it does not amount to civil rights legislation. The legislation is complex with many caveats. Oliver and Barnes (1998: 90) note: 'The Act gives only limited protection from direct discrimination . . . because not all disabled people are covered by the Act and employers and service providers are exempt if they can show that compliance would damage their business.' The Act is full of loopholes and phrases such as 'if it is reasonable' and ill-defined words like 'substantial'. Cost can be taken into account as well as health and safety regulations. It is not as robust as the Sex Discrimination Act 1975 and the Race Relations Act 1976 and has been dubbed the 'Doesn't Do Anything Act' by disabled people themselves (Trade Union Disability Alliance (TUDA) 1997). The limitations of the Act are reflected in its lack of effectiveness in the courts. Meager et al. (1999) report that, to date, 74 per cent of the cases are withdrawn or settled before a full hearing, and a further 10 per cent are dismissed.

The Act can be regarded as piecemeal legislation as large areas of life, such as education, are included only to a very limited extent, though at present the legislation is being amended to include education services. New transport has to reach minimum standards, but this applies only to land-based transport.

Within the Act, it is legal to discriminate against disabled people and discrimination can be justified, for example by employers, in ways that cannot be justified in the Sex Discrimination Act and Race Relations Act.

A major limitation of the Act was that there was no commission, that is no body to take up people's complaints. A commission, comparable to those of the Sex Discrimination Act and Race Relations Act was, however, put in place in April 2000 when the Disability Rights Commission Act 1999 established the Disability Rights Commission (DRC). At the time of writing the DRC has been in operation for just over a year, so it is early days for a full evaluation though issues have been raised. The general functions of the DRC include to work towards the elimination of discrimination against disabled persons and to promote equalization of opportunities for disabled persons (Doyle 2000). The DRC consists of no fewer than 10 and not more than 15 commissioners appointed by the Secretary of State. There is a staff of approximately 150 and a budget of £11 million. There are some early indicators of the tactics adopted by the DRC. Only 1 of the first set of 14 commissioners was a disabled activist, and conciliation and persuasion, rather than confrontation, is the main remit of the DRC (Drake 2000). Even when an organization has acted unlawfully under the DDA, the Commission can contract with the organization not to take any formal investigation if the organization undertakes not to commit any further unlawful acts of the same kind. The chairperson of the DRC has spoken of 'using the force of argument rather than the argument of force.' Persuasion, or changing people's attitudes, seems to be the DRC's main strategy. Many disabled people believe, however, that such a strategy has been the dominant official approach for many years, and has long been discredited.

In her review of the DDA Gooding (2000: 549) states: 'Perhaps what is required, above all, is a broader change to the cultural value attached to disabled people – a paradigm shift in the ways in which disability is understood.' The DDA is, in a sense, a direct expression of the politics of disability founded within a social model of disability, but remains grounded in the dominant individual/medical/tragedy model of disability.

Questions for discussion

1 In what ways might the Disability Discrimination Act play a role in promoting full participative citizenship for disabled people? What evidence is required in evaluating the effectiveness of this legislation?

2 Why are disabled people dissatisfied with the Disability Discrimination Act?

3 Mike Oliver has argued that the DRC should employ civil rights lawyers and 'sue the pants off a few really large organizations'. Would confrontation be more effective than conciliation? If so, or if not, why?

Debate activity

Debate the proposition: The priority for disabled people is the repeal, rather than strengthening, of the Disability Discrimination Act and the establishment of full Civil Rights Legislation. The following quotations may provide you with a starting point:

> The most important piece of legislation, the Disability Discrimination Act 1995, recognised the progress made by the supporters of the social model by finally introducing requirements that employers, businesses and services must ensure that all members of society have similar opportunities and are not excluded because of their disability.
>
> (Picking 2000: 17)

> the coming of the DDA put an end to the uneasy alliance between organisations of and organisations for disabled people . . . six of the main organisations for disabled people – RADAR, the National Institute for the Blind, the National Institute for the Deaf, MENCAP, MIND and SCOPE – agreed to work with the government to implement the new law. Despite protestations to the contrary by prominent representatives of these organisations, the action only served to undermine the on-going struggle for the introduction of a meaningful and effective civil rights policy.
>
> (Oliver and Barnes 1998: 90)

Further reading

Barton, L. (ed.) (2001) *Disability Politics and the Struggle for Change*. London: David Fulton.

Campbell, J. and Oliver, O. (1996) *Disability Politics: Understanding our Past, Changing our Future*. London: Routledge.

Tarrow, S. (1998) *Power in Movement: Social Movements, Collective Action and Politics*, 2nd edn. Cambridge: Cambridge University Press.

Zames Fleischer, D. and Zames, F. (2001) *The Disability Rights Movement: From Charity to Confrontation*. Philadephia, PA: Temple University Press.

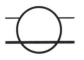

Conclusion: enabling or disabling globalization?

Rachel Hurst

(Authors' note: this book has been written to provoke and feed debates in disability studies. This conclusion is written by a well-established and respected disabled activist. It follows a similar format to previous chapters but is written as a personal statement drawing together many of the main themes of the book.)

A global world

This chapter explores the impact of globalization on the lives of disabled people. The processes of globalization have generally been detrimental to disabled people by harming or excluding them. Yet it has also stimulated the formation of international organizations of disabled people who are fighting for change (Charlton 1998). The chapter begins with a general discussion of globalization and its potential effect, for good and ill, upon the citizens of the world. The position of disabled people is then discussed and the chapter concludes with a case study of two international organizations: Disabled Peoples' International and Disability Awareness in Action.

The notion of globalization has been widely accepted. In general terms it is a multidimensional process of social change – cultural, economic and political (Cochrane and Pain 2000). It seems evident in all aspects of social life, including what we eat, our leisure pursuits and the language we use. Nevertheless, its meaning and, indeed, existence remains the subject of much dispute. Held (2000) examines three theoretical positions: globalism, traditionalism and transformationalism. Basically, globalists see globalization as a process of inevitable, irresistible and massive social change:

> National culture, economics and politics are subsumed into networks of global flows. These lessen local and national differences, autonomy and sovereignty, and produce a more homogeneous global cultures and economy.
>
> (Cochrane and Pain 2000: 22)

Traditionalists, on the other hand, resist this view and argue that global flows of money and trade around the world are not a new phenomenon. They question whether recent changes are really 'global' or just involve parts of the world. Third, transformationalists question the inevitability of the impacts of globalization. They argue for new democratic accountability in monitoring and governing change. This chapter outlines a globalist view and argues for more democratic control.

In the early 1950s, despite two world wars, most people's experience of 'abroad' and the people who lived there was extremely limited. As a young girl, the world for me was a map – much of it drawn with a red border to denote the British Empire. I read books about adventures abroad, of India and Africa, of early Chinese history, of the Renaissance and western civilization – what I knew was framed by words, pictures and a few photographs. When I first travelled to France at the age of 12, I expected it to be completely different from England, with a different language, behaviour and environment – and then I saw that they had cow parsley in the hedgerows. How could the French be so different if they had cow parsley and lived in very much the same climate and environment as we did? How could they be different if their children went to school with satchels on their backs, just as I did? My romantic dreams of difference were shattered.

Within a few years everything had changed. Television came into everybody's homes and we saw what life was really like everywhere. Travel became easier and cheaper – not only could we go to places, but also other people could travel to Britain. Increasingly the streets of London were filled with a wonderful, exciting cultural diversity. The world was no longer a map of the imagination, it was a known reality. And it was open to everyone, your back yard was no more private than the banks of the Amazon. We began to know each other's business and to want a bit of it. Trade and industry had to extend their markets worldwide to survive. National economies became dependent on exports, foreign policy was no longer just about diplomacy, flying the national flag, preventing war and maintaining pockets of Britain in a foreign land, but about commerce and the freedom of movement of people. We talked about how the world was shrinking, how international we all were. We could buy each other's foods in the supermarkets, wear each other's clothes. With satellite connections, phoning people on the other side of the world was no problem and they sounded as though they were just next door.

While we ordinary mortals were experiencing this international exchange in a directly personal way, the powerful were amassing their forces to gain control over this globe and what they felt we should hear about their activities in the media. They talked about global trade, the global economy and global warming, they stockpiled weapons against global attacks and finally they gave this internationalization a new word – globalization – a new word for a new millennium. On the positive side, there were efforts to promote justice and peace. The United Nations was founded. Eugenics, xenophobia and discrimination were outlawed through the Universal Declaration of Human Rights. Non-governmental organizations (NGOs) with objectives focused on human rights, or who directly represented disadvantaged groups, gained support and influenced the UN and other international debates.

Unfortunately, so often these efforts failed because of personal and national interests. There was much talk of rights but only a few countries made any endeavours to really implement those rights for everyone. Divisions between rich and poor grew greater and greater, even in the developed world. The Bretton Woods organizations (which include the World Bank and the International Monetary Fund) were set up after the Second World War to regulate the global economy under the direction of the United States. These organizations gained control of debt in the developing world and, along with market forces, controlled how they should trade (Thomas and Allen 2000). Non-governmental organizations were increasingly seen by the powerful as threats and barriers to what they considered was progress (Thomas 1992).

Consultation and democratic processes are words often bandied around by governments and policy makers but are hastily and loosely implemented. They are too slow for the speed required by global advancement. The powerless have become more powerless and the powerful, including the media, having a world stage to work on, have become more powerful. The greater your difference or distance from the powerful, the greater your separation from mainstream society.

So, for the person in the street, globalization has begun to mean the power of the transnational corporations and the pursuit of economic growth at huge human and environmental cost. The gap between rich and poor has widened (McGrew 2000), cutbacks and an absence of social assistance have led to increased social unrest, crime and violence as well as increased hunger, the diseases of poverty and population growth. Deregulation and the growth and power of transnationals are causing untold ecological degradation. Global forces such as trade agreements and structural adjustment policies (whereby the free market is allowed to operate with minimal state intervention) have increased hardship of local peoples and further destabilized the ecology. Local advances are swept away or ignored by global imbalances.

If that is the only potential of globalization, then we are on a path to destruction. Instead, globalization has to be a denial of all these negatives. It has to be a mechanism which allows the world to use its benefits for the good of all. Tony Blair identified in a speech in 2001 to the Labour Party Conference the real issue of globalization which is to use the global community to promote justice, to maintain rights and to ensure a world fit for everyone in which difference is seen as a gift to the world and not a deviation, and where benefits, including economic growth, are for all – not for just the few. The important factors for change must be concerted community action, justice and human rights (Blair 2001).

Questions for discussion

1 What do you understand by the term 'globalization'?
2 How far do you consider globalization to be detrimental or beneficial to the citizens of the world?
3 Who controls the processes of globalization and how is that control maintained?

The impact of globalization on disabled people

At a very basic level globalization describes the rapid flow of goods, services, people, finance and information between countries. However, most disabled people cannot even 'rapidly flow' in their own homes or communities, let alone globally (Swain et al. 1998). For them globalization is a mockery. The services and information flowing through globalization are either not relevant or accessible to disabled people or underpin, through negative attitudes, the concept that a disabled person's life is not worth living and not worth having (Charlton 1998).

Disabled people are the poorest of the poor in all countries, in terms of relative poverty in the developed world and in terms of absolute poverty in the developing world (Stone 1999b). Mainstream aid and development generally exclude disabled people (Coleridge 1993). The health status measurements of the World Health Organization (WHO 2001) see disability as a negative measurement in the same way as mortality. This leads governments to formalize that negativity in their responses to disabled people. This is done by showing no recognition of their capacity for, and rights to, full and equal participation, no recognition of the barriers that society itself has erected against that participation, and no recognition of the way in which society systematically erodes the rights of disabled people.

For disabled people the impact of globalization has been to increase our isolation, our disempowerment, emphasize our difference and demonstrate our segregation from the rest of humanity. These negative impacts have also come from: global genetic advances and assessments of our quality of life; the multinational pharmaceutical companies' hold over research, patenting and genetic advances; the invisibility of disabled people from mainstream activity and information; and the silence of our voice in the corridors of power and change. We have a long way to go before the justice needed within globalization can celebrate our difference and ensure our humanity.

In the majority of the world, disabled people are still viewed as a separate people who need special treatment and special services (Charlton 1998). Some see this separateness as the correct and appropriate response of charitable and kind people and of social and political systems based on welfare. In reality, and as confirmed by policies regarding genetic advances, the underlying assumption is that disabled people are a people whose genetic make-up should be eliminated or modified (DPI 2000). These assumptions are emphasized by world authorities such as Peter Singer, Professor of Ethics at Princeton's Center for Human Values, who stated in his 1979 book, *Practical Ethics*, that children less than 1 month old have no human consciousness and parents should be allowed to kill a severely disabled infant to end its suffering and to increase the family's happiness. Such attitudes remain prevalent today. The embryologist Bob Edwards, who worked to produce the first 'test-tube' baby, Louise Brown, recently declared that it would soon be a 'sin' to give birth to a disabled child (Rogers 1999).

These are not isolated opinions, indeed there are selective abortion laws throughout Europe that support the notion that disabled lives are not worth living. Lack of health care services, the behaviour of doctors in their treatment (or lack of it) of disabled people, the affect of cultural attitudes at the birth of disabled children and the spread of non-voluntary euthanasia practices, all underline the notion that we are dispensable. Unlike the rest of humanity, we do not have the right to life because others think our lives are not worth living. The Human Rights Violation database of Disability Awareness in Action had, by May 2001, recorded cases of violations against over 2 million disabled people. Of these cases, 21 per cent were violations of the right to life and a further 21 per cent recorded degrading or inhuman treatment.

Disabled people are invisible and ignored, not seen as people with rights. Disability is not explicitly mentioned in any of the UN Covenants and Conventions on rights and non-discrimination, except for the Convention on the Rights of the Child. Nor is it mentioned in the European Convention on Human Rights. United Nation instruments and national legislation that has been passed to support disabled people's right to freedom, dignity and non-discrimination have been systematically and universally ignored. There is rarely any compliance with the UN Standard Rules on Equalization of Opportunities for Disabled Persons, which were unanimously agreed by the UN General Assembly in 1993 (Lindqvist 2000). There are only a handful of countries (for example UK, USA, Canada, Australia, South Africa) where disabled people do have the right to non-discrimination in law and, most importantly, a means of obtaining redress. Although guidance has been provided to ensure the inclusion of disability rights in the regular monitoring of UN member states behaviour under the Covenants, the only committee that follows this guidance is the Committee on the Rights of the Child. Since January 2001, they have had regular written and verbal input from Rights for Disabled Children, an international working group to promote the situation and voice of disabled children. But this input is not financially or strategically supported by the UN. It is an initiative of disabled people's own organizations (Lansdown 2001).

Disabled people are left out of development too (Hurst 1999). While the majority of large aid agencies have policies to ensure the involvement of women in their work, very few have a policy regarding disabled people. Mainstream projects do not consider the needs of disabled people. Far too little funding is given to projects promoting social change to include disabled people or to activities run by disabled people's own organizations. Only the UN High Commission on Refugees has a policy to ensure aid goes to disabled refugees, though it is a policy that more often than not gathers dust on a top shelf rather than being put to use. Disaster relief organizations have no mechanisms to include disabled people in their strategies. Strategies and policies for the alleviation of poverty do not include disabled people. Yet, disabled people are the poorest of the poor in every country of the world with over 60 per cent of disabled people of working age being unemployed in developed countries and 297 of the 300 million disabled people in the developing world, denied access to assistance, rehabilitation, appropriate services and food (Fletcher 1995). Governments in the North sometimes include mention of disability as a cause and outcome of poverty yet they never use rights for disabled people as a criteria for debt alleviation – though they do with rights for women (Sattaur 2001).

The global information network does not address the concerns of disabled people and is generally inaccessible. Sign language is recognized as an official language in only a very few countries. Disability experience and rights are ignored or presented through negative and charitable images. For instance, coverage of the Paralympics was only a fraction of the Olympics coverage, although the athletes in many cases surpass the performance of their non-disabled counterparts, and sponsorship is non-existent. Yet some advertisers actually use disabled people like Stephen Hawkings, the leading scientist, to boost their sales.

Worst of all the voice of disabled people is generally silent in the formation of policy and absent from the structures of democracy. Only in Uganda and South Africa is there a definite strategy to ensure disabled people have a direct and democratic voice inside government. Rule 18 of the UN Standard Rules on Equalization of Opportunities for Disabled Persons specifically states the responsibility of governments to fund and involve organizations of disabled people in all policies and programmes that directly concern them, and yet this rarely happens. Disability is very low on most government agendas, is hidden within government departments and rarely has a place in mainstream policies and planning.

The provision or non-provision of benefits also isolates disabled people from mainstream society as treasuries throughout the world use disability benefits as a prime target for cuts or for accusations of fraud and an unjustified drain on exchequers. In the developing world there are no benefits for disabled people, but there is also no intention to provide them. Benefits for disabled people are seen as a waste of money. The global belief is that disabled people are unemployable, unproductive and extremely costly. However, seeing disabled people as the cost factor is not the true story. Disabled people are non-participants and non-contributory because of barriers in the environment and social attitudes and systems that disable (Russell 1998). With these barriers removed, disabled people can participate and become contributing members of society. It may mean that some may need a level of benefit and specific adjustments may have to be made – but the cost of these is minimal and offset by the cost benefits of participation. For instance, the £7 million spent by the Tyneside Underground system on becoming fully accessible was recouped within three years by profits from extra usage – not just by disabled people but by many others who found the system much more acceptable. Market economies must look to their consumers, they cannot afford to over-look the 10 per cent of the population who are disabled people. If disabled people are not able to consume, are sunk in poverty and isolation, then it is the markets that are going to suffer, as well as disabled people.

All is not doom and gloom however. The birth of Disabled Peoples' Inter-national (DPI) in 1981 is a perfect example of globalization working for jus-tice and inclusion, springing out of an oppressive form of globalization where disabled people had no voice.

Questions for discussion

1 In what ways are disabled people marginalized throughout the world?
2 What needs to be done to decrease this marginalization as globaliz-ation continues?
3 How would you sum up the commonalities and differences between disabled people throughout the world?

Coming together: international organizations of disabled people

Disabled Peoples' International grew out of confrontation between the oppressed and the powerful. In 1980, Rehabilitation International organized their world conference in Winnipeg, Canada. Rehabilitation International is an organization of professionals in disability – medical, rehabilitation and charity professionals. They organized this conference, of nearly 3000 people, to discuss how they were going to use the International Year of Disabled Per-sons that the UN had designated for 1981. Because of efforts from the few disabled people in their membership to make the organization accountable to disabled people, they invited about 200 disabled people to attend the con-ference.

These disabled individuals came from all around the world. For all of them their experience as disabled people had been hard, especially hard for those from developing countries. In fact it had been so hard and difficult that they could not imagine that things were as bad in other countries. They felt, as many people who suffer discrimination feel, that the world would not toler-ate that sort of treatment and therefore their situation, in their community, was unique – uniquely terrible.

These 200 people with their 'unique' experiences met on the first evening of the conference at a barbecue organized by the Canadian Coalition of Dis-abled People. There they quickly found that their experiences were not unique after all and that they were all systematically and daily facing discrimination and violations of their rights. This understanding of their commonality of experience gave them the unity of purpose needed to abandon the conference when they asked for and were denied a substantive voice in the proceedings. Having done so, the disabled delegates spent the next few days in workshops and meetings discussing what they should do. They decided to form an international organization of disabled people, with membership of national assemblies of disabled people of all impairments from organizations that covered all parts of each country. These national assemblies would form regional councils who would, in turn, work with the world council in producing policies and strategies for implementation. They were united in saying that the objective of this organization would be the full and equal participation of disabled people in society and comprehensive implementation of their rights. The disabled delegates finally went home to start national assemblies and a year later in Singapore, Disabled Peoples' International was born with membership from 40 countries (Driedger 1989).

There are now over 160 national assemblies, many of which represent thousands of disabled individuals of all impairments, including people with intellectual impairment. In 1992, DPI agreed that it was a human rights organization and that its membership was individually and collectively committed to global justice for disabled people. DPI is also committed to ensuring the voice of disabled people in all policies and programmes that directly effect them. 'Nothing About Us Without Us', is one of the DPI slogans. As a result DPI has had considerable influence in formulating the UN World Programme of Action Concerning Disabled Persons (1983) and the UN Standard Rules on Equalization of Opportunities for Persons with Disabilities (1993). Disabled Peoples' International is now committed to working with other international disability organizations. The purpose of this is to call for a convention on the rights of disabled people, in order to provide a global instrument that recognizes the true experience of disabled people and provides formal monitoring of member states' behaviour in implementing disability rights.

Every four years the national assemblies of DPI have an opportunity to come together in a World Assembly to share their experiences, gain strength from their unity of purpose and agree an action plan for the next four years. The action plan is, then, reviewed by regional councils for action at regional, national and local levels. DPI is unique among civil rights movements in being organized globally through a directly representative and democratic, grassroots network. The commitment to rights by the membership has led to significant social change as national assemblies consult and work with their governments to implement a rights-based approach to disability.

For the first ten years, through its democratic network, DPI began a global exchange of people, information and experience. But this exchange was mostly through the leadership. Even though these leaders worked hard to pass the information on to strengthen and empower disabled people at the grassroots and at local levels, there was little flow of information. This was seriously impeding progress in the search for justice. There were no financial and human resources to produce information in the quantities and frequency required. So in 1992, DPI came together with some of the other international disability organizations (Inclusion International, IMPACT and the World Federation of the Deaf) to set up an international information network on disability and human rights with the objective of supporting disabled people's actions at the grassroots to implement those rights. This network, Disability Awareness in Action (DAA), has produced monthly newsletters – the *Disability Tribune* – and numerous resource kits on issues of particular concern, such as organization building, consultation and influence, campaigning and working with the media. It has also produced information on the UN Standard Rules, been a decisive factor in promoting the International Day of Disabled People and is now supporting the campaign for a convention on the rights of disabled people. Disability Awareness in Action has also built up a considerable collection of evidence on the status of disabled people through examples of good practice and a database of violations against disabled people throughout the world.

Giving disabled people at the local and national level regular information has undoubtedly been welcomed and used effectively. DDA materials have been translated into over 40 national and local languages, and has influenced activities at all levels. The crucial importance of this information is that it comes from disabled people and goes to disabled people. It is not doctrinal or propaganda. It is shared experience and concrete facts. Readers are left to do with it what they will. For disabled people, whose past experience is one of isolation and oppression, this freedom is welcomed.

The global network of disabled people's organizations has grown and continues to grow. Where politically possible, organizations have influenced their government's policies and have demanded the right to choice and control over disabled individual's lives, to access public facilities, to education and employment, to life itself. They have shown that disabled people can contribute significantly to the global economy and have the right to live and participate equally, freely and fully. Through these global information and organizational networks, increasing numbers of disabled people have begun to realize that they are part of a worldwide movement – that what they do as a group in a small village in rural Africa will impact the lives of their disabled colleagues in Berlin, in the slums of Rio de Janeiro or an Indian sangha – and vice versa. In effect, they are in control of this disability globalization – not the powerful professionals or the economically strong.

The joint endeavours of DPI and DAA do provide a positive example of how effective globalization can be in the pursuit of justice for all. The evidence is clear that it is the fundamental principle of human rights that drives this effectiveness. If the experience of DPI could be replicated by others and influence global economic forces, then perhaps we could halt the present negative impacts and globalization could create a viable future for everyone, not just the few. If the fundamental principles of organization like DPI and DAA could be the shared commitment of all global activity, then perhaps globalization would not be the negative development it appears to be to so many people and could provide the justice, freedom and dignity for all that should be the pursuit of all democratic peoples.

Questions for discussion

1 Will the process of globalization ever address issues of importance to disabled people?
2 How far can organizations like DPI and DAA have an impact on the process of globalization?
3 What are the benefits of disabled people from diverse parts of the world coming together to share their experiences?

Debate activity

Debate the proposition: Globalization will be beneficial to disabled people. The following quotations may provide you with a starting point.

> There are . . . two sides to the 'permanence' of disability oppression. On one side is the capacity of oppressive structures and institutions to reproduce themselves through the myriad power relationships in everyday life. On the other side is the inevitability that oppression will generate its opposites – resistance, empowerment, and, from these, potentially, liberation and freedom.
>
> (Charlton 1998: 153)

> If we are talking about disability in the majority world then we need to talk both of survival and of social change. It does not ring true to call for better policies, provision and attitudes without also pointing to the global structures that keep millions of people locked in poverty and powerlessness. Likewise, the experience of disabled people in the minority (Western) world shows the abject failure of economic development as a stand-alone strategy for alleviating poverty or dismantling disabling barriers.
>
> (Stone 2001: 61)

Further reading

Charlton, J.I. (1998) *Nothing about Us without Us: Disability, Oppression and Empowerment.* Berkeley, CA: University of California Press.

Coleridge, P. (1993) *Disability, Liberation and Development.* Oxford: Oxfam.

Priestley, M. (ed.) (2001) *Disability and the Life Course: Global Perspectives.* Cambridge: Cambridge University Press.

Stone, E. (ed.) (1999) *Disability and Development: Learning from Action and Research in the Majority World.* Leeds: The Disability Press.

References

Abberley, P. (1993) Disabled people and normality, in J. Swain, V. Finkelstein, S. French and M. Oliver (eds) *Disabling Barriers – Enabling Environments*. London: Sage.

Abberley, P. (1999) The significance of work for the citizenship of disabled people. Paper presented at University College Dublin, 18 April, www.leeds.ac.uk.disability-studies/archive/

Abbott, P. (2000) Gender, in G. Payne (ed.) *Social Divisions*. London: Macmillan.

Abbott, P. and Meerabeau, L. (1998) Professions, professionalism and the caring professions, in P. Abbott and L. Meerabeau (eds) *The Sociology of the Caring Professions*. London: UCL Press.

Adams, J., Bornat, J. and Prickett, M. (1998) Discovering the present in stories about the past, in A. Brechin, J. Walmsley, J. Katz and S. Peace (eds) *Care Matters: Concepts, Practice and Research in Health and Social Care*. London: Sage.

Adams, J., Swain, J. and Clark, J. (2000) What's so special? Teachers' models of disability and their realisation in practice in special schools, *Disability and Society*, 15(2): 233–46.

Adams, J.E. (1998) A special environment? Learning in the MLD and SLD classroom. Unpublished PhD thesis, University of Northumbria, Newcastle upon Tyne.

Ahmad, W.I.U. (ed.) (2000) *Ethnicity, Disability and Chronic Illness*. Buckingham: Open University Press.

Ahmad, W.I.U. and Atkin, K. (eds) (1998) *Race and Community Care*. Buckingham: Open University Press.

Ahmad, W.I.U., Darr, A. and Jones, L. (2000) 'I send my child to school and he comes back an Englishman': minority ethnic deaf people, identity politics and services, in W.I.U. Ahmad (ed.) *Ethnicity, Disability and Chronic Illness*. Buckingham: Open University Press.

Albrecht, G.L., Seelman, K.D. and Bury, M. (2001) Introduction: the formation of disability studies, in G.L. Albrecht, K.D. Seelman and M. Bury (eds) *Handbook of Disability Studies*. London: Sage.

Allan, J., Brown, S. and Riddell, S. (1998) Permission to speak? Theorising special education inside the classroom, in C. Clark, A. Dyson and A. Millward (eds) *Theorising Special Education*. London: Routledge.

Allen, T. (2000) The world at war, in T. Allen and A. Thomas (eds) *Poverty and Development: Into the 21st Century*. Oxford: Oxford University Press.

Alston, P. (1999) A framework for the comparative analysis of bills of rights, in P. Alston (ed.) *Promoting Human Rights through Bills of Rights: Comparative Perspectives*. Oxford: Oxford University Press.

Andrews, J. with Rolph, S. (2000) Scrub, scrub, scrub . . . bad times and good times: some of the jobs I've had in my life, in D. Atkinson, M. McCarthy, J. Walmsley et al. (eds) *Good Times, Bad Times: Women with Learning Difficulties Telling their Stories*. Kidderminster: British Institute of Learning Disabilities.

Armstrong, F., Belmont, B. and Verillon, A. (2000) 'Vive la differance?' Exploring context, policy and change in special education in France: developing cross-cultural collaboration, in F. Armstrong and L. Barton (eds) *Inclusive Education: Policy, Contexts and Comparative Perspectives*. London: David Fulton.

Asch, A. (2001) Disability, bioethics and human rights, in G.L. Albrecht, K.D. Seelman and M. Bury (eds) *Handbook of Disability Studies*. London: Sage.

Aspis, S. (1999) What they don't tell people with learning difficulties, in M. Corker and S. French (eds) *Disability Discourse*. Buckingham: Open University Press.

Atkinson, D. (1999) *Advocacy: A Review*. York: Joseph Rowntree Foundation.

Baily, M.A. (2000) Why I had an amniocentesis, in E. Parens and A. Asch (eds) *Prenatal Testing and Disability Rights*. Washington, DC: Georgetown University Press.

Baker, M. (1991) *With All Hopes Dashed in the Human Zoo*. Warminster: Danny Howell.

Banton, M. and Hirsch, M.M. (2000) *Double Invisibility: Report on Research into the Needs of Black Disabled People in Coventry*. Warwick: Warwickshire County Council.

Barnes, C. (1991) *Disabled People in Britain and Discrimination*. London: Hurst in association with the British Council of Organizations of Disabled People.

Barnes, C. (1994) Images of disability, in S. French (ed.) *On Equal Terms: Working with Disabled People*. Oxford: Butterworth: Heinemann.

Barnes, C. (1998) The social model of disability: a sociological phenomenon ignored by sociologists, in T. Shakespeare (ed.) *The Disability Reader: Social Science Perspectives*. London: Cassell.

Barnes, C. and Mercer, G. (1995) Disability: emancipation, community participation and disabled people, in G. Craig and M. Mayo (eds) *Community Empowerment: A Reader in Participation and Development*. London: Zed Books.

Barnes, C. and Mercer, G. (eds) (1996) *Exploring the Divide: Illness and Disability*. Leeds: The Disability Press.

Barnes, C. and Mercer, G. (2001a) The politics of disability and the struggle for change, in L. Barton (ed.) *Disability Politics and the Struggle for Change*. London: David Fulton.

Barnes, C. and Mercer, G. (2001b) Disability culture: assimilation or inclusion? in G.L. Abrecht, K.D. Seelman and M. Bury (eds) *Handbook of Disability Studies*. London: Sage.

Barnes, C. and Mercer, M. (1997) *Doing Disability Research*. Leeds: The Disability Press.

Barnes, C. and Oliver, M. (1995) Disability rights: rhetoric and reality in the UK, *Disability and Society*, 10(4): 111–16.

Barnes, C., Mercer, M. and Shakespeare, T. (1999) *Exploring Disability: A Sociological Introduction*. Cambridge: Polity Press.

Barnes, M. and Bowl, R. (2000) *Taking over the Asylum: Empowerment and Mental Health*. Basingstoke: Palgrave.

Bartlett, J. (1994) *Will You Be Mother? Women Who Choose to Say No*. London: Virago.

Barton, L. (1996) Sociology and disability: some emerging issues, in L. Barton (ed.) *Disability and Society: Emerging Issues and Insights*. London: Longman.

Barton, L. (1997) The politics of special educational needs, in L. Barton and M. Oliver (eds) *Disability Studies: Past, Present and Future*. Leeds: The Disability Press.

Barton, L. (2001) Disability, struggle and the politics of hope, in L. Barton (ed.) *Disability Politics and the Struggle for Change*. London: David Fulton.

Basnett, I. (2001) Health care professionals and their attitudes towards and decisions affecting disabled people, in G.L. Albrecht, K.D. Seelman and M. Bury (eds) *Handbook of Disability Studies*. London: Sage.

Bauman, Z. (1997) *Thinking Sociologically*. Oxford: Blackwell.

Baxter, C. (1995) Confronting colour blindness: developing better services for people with learning disabilities from black and ethnic minority communities, in T. Philpot and L. Ward (eds) *Values and Visions: Changing Ideas for Services for People with Learning Disabilities*. Oxford: Butterworth: Heinemann.

Baynton, D.C. (1996) *American Culture and the Campaign against Sign Language*. Chicago: University of Chicago Press.

Baynton, D.C. (2001) Disability and the justification of inequality in American history, in P.K. Longmore and L. Umansky (eds) *The New Disability History: American Perspectives*. New York: New York University Press.

Becker, S. (1997) *Responding to Poverty: The Politics of Cash and Care*. London: Longman.

Begum, N. (1994a) Mirror, mirror on the wall, in N. Begum, M. Hill and A. Stevens (eds) *Reflections: Views of Black Disabled People on their Lives and Community Care*. London: Central Council for Education and Training in Social Work.

Begum, N. (1994b) Snow White, in L. Keith (ed.) *Mustn't Grumble: Writing by Disabled Women*. London: The Women's Press.

Begum, N. (1996) Doctor, doctor . . .: disabled women's experiences of general practitioners, in J. Morris (ed.) *Encounters with Strangers: Feminism and Disability*. London: The Women's Press.

Beresford, P. and Wilson, A. (1998) Social exclusion and social work: challenging the contradictions of exclusive debate, in M. Barry and C. Hallett (eds) *Social Exclusion and Social Work: Issues of Theory, Policy and Practice*. Lyme Regis: Russell House.

Beveridge, W. (1948) *Voluntary Action: A Report on Methods of Social Advance*. London: Allen & Unwin.

Bhavnani, R. (1994) *Black Women in the Labour Market: A Research Review*. Manchester: Equal Opportunities Commission.

Bignall, T. and Butt, J. (2000) *Between Ambition and Achievement: Young Black Disabled People's Views and Experiences of Independence and Independent Living*. Bristol: Policy Press.

Blair, T. (2001) Speech at Labour Party Conference, 2 October.

Boazman, S. (1999) Inside aphasia, in C. Corker and S. French (eds) *Disability Discourse*. Buckingham: Open University Press.

Bracking, S. (1993) An introduction to the idea of independent integrated living: a brief overview, in C. Barnes (ed.) *Making our Own Choices: Independent Living, Personal Assistance and Disabled People*. Belper: British Council of Organizations of Disabled People.

Bradley, H. (1996) *Fractured Identities: Changing Patterns of Inequality*. Cambridge: Polity Press.

Brechin, A. (1998) Introduction, in A. Brechin, J. Walmsley, J. Katz and S. Peace (eds) *Care Matters: Concepts, Practice and Research in Health and Social Care*. London: Sage.

Brechin, A. (1999) Understandings of learning disability, in J. Swain and S. French (eds) *Therapy and Learning Difficulties: Advocacy, Participation and Partnership*. Oxford: Butterworth-Heinemann.

Brechin, A. (2000) The challenge of caring relationships, in A. Brechin, H. Brown and M.A. Eby (eds) *Critical Practice in Health and Social Care*. London: Sage.

Brigham, L., Atkinson, D., Jackson, M., Rolph, S. and Walmsley, J. (2000) *Crossing Boundaries: Change and Continuity in the History of Learning Disability.* Kidderminster: British Institute of Learning Disabilities.

British Dyslexia Association (2002) http://www.bda-dyslexia.org.uk

British Medical Association (Steering Group on Human Genetics) (1998) *Human Genetics: Choice and Responsibility.* Oxford: Oxford University Press.

British Organisation of Non-Parents (BON) (undated) *You Do Have a Choice!* London: BON.

Brown, G. and Atkins, M. (1988) *Effective Teaching in Higher Education.* London: Methuen.

Burden, T. and Hamm, T. (2000) Responding to socially excluded groups, in J. Percy-Smith (ed.) *Policy Responses to Social Exclusion: Towards Inclusion?* Buckingham: Open University Press.

Burr, V. (1997) *An Introduction to Social Constructionism.* London: Routledge.

Butt, J. and Box, L. (1997) *Supportive Services, Effective Strategies: The Views of Black-Led Organizations and Social Care Agencies on the Future of Social Care for Black Communities.* London: Race Equality Unit.

Butt, J. and Mirza, K. (1996) *Social Care and Black Communities.* London: Race Equality Unit.

Butt, J., Bignall, T. and Stone, E. (2000) *Directing Support: Report from a Workshop on Direct Payments and Black and Minority Ethnic Disabled People.* York: Joseph Rowntree Foundation.

Campbell, J. and Oliver, M. (1996) *Disability Politics: Understanding our Past, Changing our Future.* London: Routledge.

Campbell, P. (1996) The history of the user movement in the United Kingdom, in T. Heller, J. Reynolds, R. Gomm, R. Muston and S. Pattison (eds) *Mental Health Matters: A Reader.* London: Macmillan.

Campling, J. (ed.) (1981) *Images of Ourselves: Women with Disabilities Talking.* London: Routledge and Kegan Paul.

Carr, L. (2000) Enabling our destruction?, *Coalition*, August: 29–36.

Cassidy, B., Lord, R. and Mandell, N. (1995) Silenced and forgotten women: race, poverty and disability, in N. Mandell (ed.) *Feminist Issues: Race, Class and Sexuality.* Scarborough, Ontario: Prentice Hall.

Castle, W.E., Coulter, J.M., Davenport, C.B., East, E.M., and Tower, W.L. (1912) *Heredity and Eugenics: A Course of Lectures Summarising Recent Advances in Knowledge in Variation, Heredity, and Evolution and its Relation to Plant, Animal, and Human Improvement and Welfare.* Chicago: University of Chicago Press.

Charlton, J.I. (1998) *Nothing about Us without Us: Disability, Oppression and Empowerment.* Berkeley, CA: University of California Press.

Clarke, J. and Cochrane, A. (1998) The social construction of social problems, in E. Saraga (ed.) *Embodying the Social: Constructions of Difference.* London: Routledge.

Clough, P. and Barton, L. (eds) (1995) *Making Difficulties: Research and the Construction of Special Educational Needs.* London: Paul Chapman.

Cochrane, A. and Pain, K. (2000) A globalizing society?, in D. Held (ed.) *A Globalizing World? Culture, Economics, Politics.* London: Routledge.

Coleridge, P. (1993) *Disability, Liberation and Development.* Oxford: Oxfam.

Connect (2001) *'Whole People . . . talk here'*, First Annual Review. London: Connect.

Contact a Family (CaF) (2001) http://www.cafamily.org.uk

Cook, T. and Swain, J. (2001) Parents' perspectives on the closure of a special school: towards inclusion in partnership, *Educational Review*, 53(2): 191–8.

Cook, T., Swain, J. and French, S. (2001) Voices from segregated schooling: towards an inclusive education system, *Disability and Society*, 16(2): 293–310.

Cooper, J. and Vernon, S. (1996) *Disability and the Law*. London: Jessica Kingsley.

Corbett, J. (1991) 'So, who wants to be normal?', *Disability, Handicap and Society*, 6(3): 259–60.

Corbett, J. (1996) *Bad-Mouthing: The Language of Special Needs*. London: Falmer.

Corbett, J. and Ralph, S. (1994) Empowering adults: the changing imagery of charity advertising, *Australian Disability Review*, 1: 5–14.

Corker, M. (1996) *Deaf Transitions: Images and Origins of Deaf Families, Deaf Communities and Deaf Identities*. London: Jessica Kingsley.

Corker, M. and French, S. (eds) (1999) *Disability Discourse*. Buckingham: Open University Press.

Cross, M. (1998) *Proud Child, Safer Child: A Handbook for Parents and Carers of Disabled Children*. London: The Women's Press.

Crow, L. (1996) Including all of our lives: renewing the social model of disability, in J. Morris (ed.) *Encounters with Strangers: Feminism and Disability*. London: The Women's Press.

Crow, L. (2000) Helen Keller: re-thinking the problematic icon, *Disability and Society*, 15(6): 845–59.

Daunt, P. (1991) *Meeting Disability: A European Response*. London: Cassell.

Davies, C. (1998) The cloak of professionalism, in M. Allott and M. Robb (eds) *Understanding Health and Social Care: An Introductory Reader*. London: Sage.

Davies, C. (1999) Caring for health, in *Understanding Health and Social Care*. Open University Course (K100), Block 1, Unit 2. Milton Keynes: The Open University.

Davis, K. (1993) The crafting of good clients, in J. Swain, V. Finkelstein, S. French and M. Oliver (eds) *Disabling Barriers – Enabling Environments*. London: Sage.

Davis, L.J. (1995) *Enforcing Normalcy: Disability, Deafness and the Body*. London: Verso.

Davis, L.J. (1997) Constructing normalcy: the bell curve, the novel and the invention of the disabled body in the nineteenth century, in L.J. Davis (ed.) *The Disability Studies Reader*. London: Routledge.

Dawson, C. (2000) *Independent Successes: Implementing Direct Payments*. York: Joseph Rowntree Foundation.

Degener, T. (1995) Disabled persons and human rights: the legal framework, in T. Degener and Y. Koster (eds) *Human Rights and Disabled Persons: Essays and Relevant Human Rights Instruments*. Dortrecht: Martinus Nijhoff.

Department for Education and Employment (DfEE) (1997) *Excellence for All Children: Meeting Special Educational Needs*. London: HMSO.

Department for Education and Employment (DfEE) (2000a) *SEN Code of Practice on the Identification and Assessment of Pupils with Special Education Needs*. London: DfEE.

Department for Education and Employment (DfEE) (2000b) *Statistics of Education: Special Education Needs January 2000, 09/00*. London: DfEE.

Department of Social Security (1999) *Opportunity for All: Tackling Poverty and Social Exclusion*, Cm 4445. London: HMSO.

Disability Rights Task Force (1999) *From Exclusion to Inclusion: A Report of the Disability Rights Task Force on Civil Rights for Disabled People*. London: Department for Education and Employment.

Disabled Peoples' International (DPI) (2000) Disabled people speak on the new genetics. Geneva: DPI.

Doyal, L. (1998) The new obstetrics: science or social control?, in M. Allott and M. Robb (eds) *Understanding Health and Social Care*. London: Sage.

Doyal, L. and Gough, I. (1991) *A Theory of Human Need*. London: Macmillan.

Doyle, B.J. (2000) *Disability Discrimination: Law and Practice*, 3rd edn. Bristol: Jordan.

Drake, R.F. (1996a) A critique of the role of traditional charities, in L. Barton (ed.) *Disability and Society: Emerging Issues and Insights*. London: Longman.

Drake, R.F. (1996b) Charities, authority and disabled people: a qualitative study, *Disability and Society*, 11(1): 5–23.

Drake, R. (1999) *Understanding Disability Policy*. London: Macmillan.

Drake, R. (2000) Disabled people, new Labour, benefits and work, *Critical Social Policy*, 20(4): 421–39.

Driedger, D. (1989) *The Last Civil Rights Movement*. London: Hurst.

Dyslexia Institute (2002) http://www.dyslexia-inst.org.uk

Easton, A. (1996) Introduction: what is women's studies?, in T. Cosslett, A. Easton and P. Summerfield (eds) *Women, Power and Resistance: An Introduction to Women's Studies*. Buckingham: Open University Press.

Ellis, K. (1993) *Squaring the Circle: User and Carer Participation in Needs Assessment*. York: Joseph Rowntree Foundation.

Etheridge, D.T. and Mason, H.L. (1994) *The Visually Impaired: Curriculum Access and Entitlement in Further Education*. London: David Fulton.

Evans, R. and Banton, M. (2001) *Learning from Experience: Involving Black Disabled People in Shaping Services*. Leamington Spa: Council of Disabled People, Warwickshire.

Fagan, T. and Lee, P. (1997) New social movements and social policy: a case study of the disability movement, in M. Lavalette and A. Pratt (eds) *Social Policy: A Conceptual and Theoretical Introduction*. London: Sage.

Fawcett, B. (2000) *Feminist Perspectives on Disability*. Harlow: Pearson Educational.

Featherstone, M. (1991) The body in consumer culture, in M. Featherstone, M. Hepworth and B.S. Turner (eds) *The Body: Social Process and Cultural Theory*. London: Sage.

Finkelstein, V. (1991) Disability: an administrative challenge? (The health and welfare heritage), in M. Oliver (ed.) *Social Work: Disabled People and Disabling Environments*. London: Jessica Kingsley.

Finkelstein, V. (1996) Outside, 'Inside Out', *Coalition*, April: 12.

Finkelstein, V. (1998) Emancipating disability studies, in T. Shakespeare (ed.) *The Disability Reader: Social Science Perspectives*. London: Cassell.

Finkelstein, V. (2001) A personal journey into disability politics. Paper given at Leeds University Centre for Disability Studies, 7 February. www.leeds.ac.uk/disability_studies/links.htm

Finkelstein, V. and Stuart, O. (1996) Developing new services, in G. Hales (ed.) *Beyond Disability: Towards an Enabling Society*. London: Sage.

Finlay, L. (2000) The challenge of professionalism, in A. Brechin, H. Brown and M.A. Eby (eds) *Critical Practice in Health and Social Care*. London: Sage.

Fiske, J. (1993) *Power Plays, Power Works*. London: Verso.

Fletcher, A. (1995) *Overcoming Obstacles to the Integration of Disabled People*. London: Disability Awareness in Action.

Foreman, M. (1999a) Women made vulnerable, in M. Foreman (ed.) *AIDS and Men: Taking Risks or Taking Responsibility*. London: Panos Institute and Zed Books.

Foreman, M. (ed.) (1999b) *AIDS and Men: Taking Risks or Taking Responsibility*. London: Panos Institute and Zed Books.

Foucault, M. (1980) The eye of power, in C. Gordon (ed.) *Power/Knowledge: Selected Interviews and Other Writings 1973–1977 by Michel Foucault*. Brighton: Harvester.

French, S. (1989) Mind your language, *Nursing Times*, 85(2): 29–31.

French, S. (1993a) What's so great about independence?, in J. Swain, V. Finkelstein, S. French and M. Oliver (eds) *Disabling Barriers – Enabling Environments*. London: Sage.

French, S. (1993b) Setting a record straight, in J. Swain, V. Finkelstein, S. French and M. Oliver (eds) *Disabling Barriers – Enabling Environments*. London: Sage.

French, S. (1996) Out of sight, out of mind: the experience and effects of a 'special' residential school, in J. Morris (ed.) *Encounters with Strangers: Feminism and Disability*. London: The Women's Press.

French, S. (1997) Society and the changing nature of illness and disease, in S. French (ed.) *Physiotherapy: A Psychosocial Approach*, 2nd edn. Oxford: Butterworth-Heinemann.

French, S. (2001) *Disabled People and Employment: A Study of the Working Lives of Visually Impaired Physiotherapists*. Aldershot: Ashgate.

French, S. and Sim, J. (1993) *Writing: A Guide for Therapists*. Oxford: Butterworth-Heinemann.

French, S. and Swain, J. (1999) Conclusion: reflections on therapy and learning difficulties, in J. Swain and S. French (eds) *Therapy and Learning Difficulties: Advocacy, Participation and Partnership*. Oxford: Butterworth-Heinemann.

French, S. and Swain, J. (2000) Personal perspectives on the experience of exclusion, in M. Moore (ed.) *Insider Perspectives on Inclusion: Raising Voices, Raising Issues*. Sheffield: Philip Armstrong.

French, S. and Swain, J. (2001) The relationship between disabled people and health and welfare professionals, in G.L. Albrecht, K.D. Seelman and M. Bury (eds) *Handbook of Disability Studies*. London: Sage.

French, S. and Swain, J. (2002) Across the disability divide: whose tragedy?, in K.W.M. Fulford, D.L. Dickenson and T.H. Murray (eds) *Healthcare Ethics and Human Values*. Oxford: Blackwell.

French, S., Neville, S. and Laing, J. (1994) *Teaching and Learning: A Guide for Therapists*. Oxford: Butterworth-Heinemann.

French, S., Gillman, M. and Swain J. (1997) *Working with Visually Disabled People: Bridging Theory and Practice*. Birmingham: Venture Press.

Freund, P.E.S. and McGuire, M.B. (1995) *Health, Illness and the Social Body: A Critical Sociology*, 2nd edn. Englewood Cliffs, NJ: Prentice Hall.

Friere, P. (1996) *Pedagogy of the Oppressed*. Harmondsworth: Penguin.

Fromm, E. (1984) *To Have or To Be*. London: Abacus.

Fromm, E. (2001) *The Fear of Freedom*. London: Routledge.

Frost, L. (2001) *Young Women and the Body: A Feminist Sociology*. Basingstoke: Palgrave.

Fulcher, J. and Scott, J. (1999) *Sociology*. Oxford: Oxford University Press.

Garland Thomson, R. (1997) *Extraordinary Bodies: Figuring Physical Disability in American Culture and Literature*. New York: Columbia University Press.

Genesis (the book of) (1964) *The Thompson Chain-Reference Bible*. London: Eyre and Spottiswoode.

Gerard, D. (1983) *Charities in Britain: Conservatism or Change?* London: Bedford Square Press.

Gillespie, M.A. (1998) Mirror, mirror, in R. Weitz (ed.) *The Politics of Women's Bodies: Sexuality, Appearance and Behaviour*. Oxford: Oxford University Press.

Gillespie-Sells, K., Hill, M. and Robbins, B. (1998) *She Dances to Different Drums: Research into Disabled Women's Sexuality*. London: King's Fund.

Gillman, M., Swain, J. and Heyman, B. (1997) Life history or 'case' history: the objectification of people with learning difficulties through the tyranny of professional discourses, *Disability and Society*, 12(5): 675–93.

Gillman, M., Heyman, B. and Swain, J. (2000) What's in a name? The implications of diagnosis for people with learning difficulties and their family carers, *Disability and Society*, 15(3): 389–409.

Giugni, M., McAdam, D. and Tilly, C. (eds) (1999) *How Social Movements Matter*. Minneapolis, MN: University of Minnesota Press.

Gleeson, B.J. (1997) Disability studies: a historical materialist view, *Disability and Society*, 12(2): 1179–202.

Glover, D. and Strawbridge, S. (1985) *The Sociology of Knowledge*. Ormskirk: Causeway.

Goffman, E. (1976) *The Presentation of Self in Everyday Life*. Harmondsworth: Penguin.

Gomm, R. (1999) Information and involvement, in *Understanding Health and Social Care* (K100), Open University Course, Block 6, Unit 22. Milton Keynes: The Open University.

Gooding, C. (1996) *Blackstone's Guide to the Disability Discrimination Act 1995*. London: Blackstone Press Ltd.

Gooding, C. (2000) Disability Discrimination Act: from statute to practice, *Critical Social Policy*, 20(4): 533–49.

Gosling, V. and Cotterill, L. (2000) An employment project as a route to social inclusion for people with learning difficulties?, *Disability and Society*, 15(7): 1001–18.

Gough, I. (1998) What are human needs?, in J. Franklin (ed.) *Social Policy and Social Justice*. Cambridge: Polity Press.

Gray, A. (2001) *Lanark*, Vol. 1, Book 3. Edinburgh: Cannongate.

Gray, J. (2000) Inclusion: a radical critique, in P. Askonas and A. Stewart (eds) *Social Inclusion: Possibilities and Tensions*. New York: St Martin's Press.

Grieve, G.P. (1988) Clinical examination and the SOAP mnemonic, *Physiotherapy*, 74(2): 97.

Griffin, G. (1998) Uneven development – women's studies in higher education in the 1990s, in D. Malina and S. Maslin-Prothero (eds) *Surviving the Academy: Feminist Perspectives*. London: Falmer.

Groce, N.E. (1985) *Everyone Here Spoke Sign Language: Hereditary Deafness on Martha's Vineyard*. Cambridge, MA: Harvard University Press.

Gross, R.D. (1987) *Psychology: The Science of Mind and Behaviour*. London: Edward Arnold.

Guardian, The (2001) Ministers to tackle £6bn incapacity benefit bill, 4 July.

Habeshaw, S., Habeshaw, T. and Gibbs, G. (1988) *53 Interesting Things to Do in your Seminars and Tutorials*. Bristol: Technical and Educational Services.

Hall, S. (1990) Cultural identity and Diaspora, in J. Rutherford (ed.) *Identity: Community, Culture and Difference*. London: Lawrence and Wishart.

Ham, C. (1999) *Health Policy in Britain*, 4th edn. Basingstoke: Palgrave.

Hancock, P., Hughes, B., Jagger, E. et al. (2000) *The Body, Culture and Society: An Introduction*. Buckingham: Open University Press.

Hanvey, C. and Philpot, T. (eds) (1996) *Sweet Charity: The Role and Workings of Voluntary Organizations*. London: Routledge.

Harris, M., Rochester, C. and Halfpenny, P. (2001) Voluntary organisations and social policy: twenty years of change, in M. Harris and C. Rochester (eds) *Voluntary Organisations and Social Policy in Britain: Perspectives on Change and Choice*. Basingstoke: Palgrave.

Harrison, T. (1987) *Selected Poems*. Harmondsworth: Penguin.

Hasler, F., Campbell, J. and Zarb, G. (1999) *Direct Routes to Independence: A Guide to Local Authority Implementation and Management of Direct Payments*. London: Policy Studies Institute.

Hatt, S. (2000) The different worlds of work, in G. Dawson and S. Hatt (eds) *Market, State and Feminism: The Economics of Feminist Policy*. Aldershot: Edward Elgar.

Held, D. (ed.) (2000) *A Globalizing World? Culture, Economics, Politics*. London: Routledge in association with The Open University.

Hetherington, K. (1998) *Expressions of Identity: Space, Performance, Politics*. London: Sage.

Hevey, D. (1992) *The Creatures that Time Forgot: Photography and Disability Imagery*. London: Routledge.

Hewitt, T. and Smyth, I. (2000) Is the world overpopulated?, in T. Allen and A. Thomas (eds) *Poverty and Development: Into the 21ˢᵗ Century*. Oxford: Oxford University Press.

Hill, M. (1994) 'They are not our brothers': the disability movement and the black disability movement, in N. Begum, M. Hill and A. Stevens (eds) *Reflections: Views of Black Disabled People on their Lives and Community Care*. London: Central Council for Education and Training in Social Work.

Hill-Collins, P. (1990) *Black Feminist Thought: Knowledge, Consciousness and the Politics of Empowerment*. Oxford: Unwin-Heinemann.

Ho, M.W. (1999) *Genetic Engineering: Dream or Nightmare?* Dublin: Gateway.

Hoggart, R. (1995) *The Way We Live Now*. London: Chatto and Windus.

Holliday Willey, L. (1999) *Pretending to be Normal: Living with Asperger's Syndrome*. London: Jessica Kingsley.

Holman, A. with Bewley, C. (1999) *Funding Freedom 2000: People with Learning Difficulties Using Direct Payments*. London: Values into Action.

Hughes, G. (1998) A suitable case for treatment? Constructions of disability, in E. Saraga (ed.) *Embodying the Social: Constructions of Difference*. London: Routledge.

Hugman, R. (1991) *Power in Caring Professions*. London: Macmillan.

Hull, J.M. (1991) *Touching the Rock: An Experience of Blindness*. London: Arrow.

Hull, J.M. (1997) *On Sight and Insight: A Journey into the World of Blindness*. Oxford: Oneworld.

Humphries, S. and Gordon, P. (1992) *Out of Sight: The Experience of Disability 1900–1950*. Plymouth: Northcote House.

Hurst, R. (1999) Disabled people's organisations and development: strategies for change, in E. Stone (ed.) *Disability and Development: Learning from Action and Research in the Majority World*. Leeds: The Disability Press.

Hyde, M. (2000) From welfare to work? Social policy for disabled people of working age in the United Kingdom in the 1990s, *Disability and Society*, 15(2): 327–41.

Illich, I. (1977) Disabling professions, in I. Illich, I.K. Zola, J. McKnight, J. Caplan and H. Shaiken (eds) *Disabling Professions*. London: Marion Boyars.

Jacobus, M., Fox Keller, E. and Shuttleworth, S. (eds) (1990) *Body/Politics: Women and the Discourses of Science*. London: Routledge.

Jenkins, R. (1996) *Social Identity*. London: Routledge.

Johnson, J. (1998) The emergence of care as a policy, in A. Brechin, J. Walmsley, J. Katz and S. Peace (eds) *Care Matters: Concepts, Practice and Research in Health and Social Care*. London: Sage.

Johnson, R. (1993) 'Attitudes don't just hang in the air . . .' : disabled people's perceptions of physiotherapists, *Physiotherapy*, 79(9): 619–26.

Jones, A. (1992) Civil rights, citizenship and the welfare agenda for the 1990s, in National Institute for Social Work. *Who Owns Welfare?* London: National Institute for Social Work.

Jones, C. (1983) *State Social Work and the Working Class*. London: Macmillan.

Jones, L., Atkin, K. and Ahmad, W.I.U. (2001) Supporting Asian deaf young people and their families: the role of professionals and services, *Disability and Society*, 16(1): 51–70.

Kalekin-Fishman, K. (2001) The hidden injuries of a slight limp, in M. Priestley (ed.) *Disability and the Life Course*. Cambridge: Cambridge University Press.

Kaw, E. (1998) Medicalisation of racial features: Asian-American women and plastic surgery, in R. Weitz (ed.) *The Politics of Women's Bodies: Sexuality, Appearance and Behaviour*. Oxford: Oxford University Press.

Kealey, T. (2000) Don't blame eugenics, blame politics, *Galton Institute Newsletter*, June: 7.

Keith, L. (1994) Tomorrow I'm going to rewrite the English language, in L. Keith (ed.) *Mustn't Grumble: Writing by Disabled Women*. London: The Women's Press.

Keith, L. (2001) *Take Up thy Bed and Walk: Death, Disability and Cure in Classic Fiction for Girls*. London: The Women's Press.

Keith, L. and Morris, J. (1995) Easy targets: a disability rights perspective on the 'Children as Carers' debate, *Critical Social Policy*, 15(2): 36–57.

Kendall, J. and Knapp, M. (1995) A loose and baggy monster; boundaries, definitions and typologies, in J. Davis Smith, C. Rochester and R. Hedley (eds) *An Introduction to the Voluntary Sector*. London: Routledge.

Kent, D. (2000) Somewhere a mocking bird, in E. Parens and A. Asch (eds) *Prenatal Testing and Disability Rights*. Washington, DC: Georgetown University Press.

Kevles, D. (1999) *In the Name of Eugenics: Genetics and the Uses of Human Heredity*. Cambridge, MA: Harvard University Press.

Langford, W. (1996) Romantic love and power, in T. Cosslett, A. Easton and P. Summerfield (eds) *Women, Power and Resistance: An Introduction to Women's Studies*. Buckingham: Open University Press.

Lansdown, G. (2001) *It is our World*. London: Disability Awareness in Action.

Lawler, S. (1996) Motherhood and identity, in T. Cosslett, A. Easton and P. Summerfield (eds) *Women, Power and Resistance: An Introduction to Women's Attitudes*. Buckingham: Open University Press.

Lawrence, P. and Swain, J. (1997) Sexuality and disability, in S. French (ed.) *Physiotherapy: A Psychosocial Approach*, 2nd edn. Oxford: Butterworth-Heinemann.

Legesse, A. (1980) Human rights in African political culture, in K.W. Thompson (ed.) *The Moral Imperatives of Human Rights: A World Survey*. Washington, DC: University Press of America.

LeVay, S. (1993) *The Sexual Brain*. Cambridge, MA: Massachusetts Institute of Technology Press.

Levitas, R. (1996) The concept of social exclusion and the new Durkheimian hegemony, *Critical Social Policy*, 16(1): 5–20.

Lewis, G. (ed.) (1998) *Forming Nation, Framing Welfare*. London: Routledge.

Lewis, G. (2002) *Social Construction and the Study of Social Policy: An Introduction to D218*. Milton Keynes: The Open University.

Lindqvist, B. (2000) Fundamental rights of disabled persons consistently violated around world, Commission for Social Development, SOC/4528, *Special Rapporteur of the UN Commission for Social Development*, www.un.org/pubs/index.html

Linton, S. (1998a) Disability studies/not disability studies, *Disability and Society*, 13(4): 525–40.

Linton, S. (1998b) *Claiming Disability: Knowledge and Identity*. New York: New York University Press.

Lloyd, M. (1992) 'Does she boil eggs?' Towards a feminist model of disability, *Disability, Handicap and Society*, 7(3): 207–21.

Locke, M., Robson, P. and Howlett, S. (2001) Users: at the centre or the sidelines?, in M. Harris and C. Rochester (eds) *Voluntary Organisations and Social Policy in Britain: Perspectives on Change and Choice*. Basingstoke: Palgrave.

Lonsdale, S. (1990) *Women and Disability: The Experience of Women with Disability.* London: Macmillan.

Lorde, A. (1984) *Sister Outsider.* Freedom, CA: Crossing Press.

Loxley, A. and Thomas, G. (1997) From inclusive policy to exclusive real world: an international review, *Disability and Society*, 12(2): 273–91.

Lumb, K. (2000) Editorial comment, *Coalition*, August: 4.

McAdam, D. (1994) Culture and social movements, in E. Larana, H. Johnston and J.R. Gusfield (eds) *New Social Movements: From Ideology to Identity.* Philadelphia, PA: Temple University Press.

McAllister, F. with Clarke, L. (1998) *Choosing Childlessness.* London: Family Studies Centre.

McColl, M.A. and Bickenbach, J.E. (1998) *Introduction to Disability.* London: W.B. Saunders.

McCoy, L. (1998) Education for labour: social problems of nationhood, in G. Lewis (ed.) *Forming Nation, Framing Welfare.* London: Routledge.

Macfarlane, A. (1996) Aspects of intervention: consultation, care, help and support, in G. Hales (ed.) *Beyond Disability: Towards an Enabling Society.* London: Sage.

McGrew, A. (2000) Sustainable globalisation? The global politics of development and exclusion in the new world order, in T. Allen and A. Thomas (eds) *Poverty and Development: Into the 21st Century.* Oxford: Oxford University Press.

McKnight, J. (1981) Professional service and disabling help, in A. Brechin, P. Liddiard and J. Swain (eds) *Handicap in a Social World.* Sevenoaks: Hodder and Stoughton in association with The Open University.

McKnight, J. (1995) *The Careless Society: Community and its Counterfeits.* New York: Basic Books.

McLaren, P. and Leonard, P. (1993) *Paulo Freire: A Critical Encounter.* London: Routledge.

McNally, S.J. (1997) Representation, in B. Gates (ed.) *Learning Disabilities.* Edinburgh: Churchill Livingstone.

Marshall, G. (ed.) (1998) *Oxford Dictionary of Sociology.* Oxford: Oxford University Press.

Marx, K. (1955) *The Poverty of Philosophy.* Moscow: Progress.

Marx, K. and Engels, F. (1968) *Selected Works.* London: Lawrence and Wishart.

Maslow, A. (1954) *Motivation and Personality*, 2nd edn. London: Harper and Row.

Mason, M. (1992) Internalised oppression, in R. Rieser and M. Mason (eds) *Disability Equality in the Classroom: A Human Rights Issues.* London: Disability Equality in Education.

Mason, M. (2000) *Incurably Human.* London: Working Press.

May, D. (2000) Becoming adult: school leaving, jobs and the transition to adult life, in D. May (ed.) *Transition and Change in the Lives of People with Intellectual Disabilities.* London: Jessica Kingsley.

Meager, N., Dole, B., Evans, C. et al. (1999) *Monitoring the Disability Discrimination Act (1995).* London: Department for Education and Employment.

Meekosha, H. (1998) Body battles: bodies, gender and disability, in T. Shakespeare (ed.) *The Disability Reader: Social Science Perspectives.* London: Cassell.

Middleton, L. (1997) *The Art of Assessment.* Birmingham: Venture Press.

Middleton, L. (1999) *Disabled Children: Challenging Social Exclusion.* Oxford: Blackwell.

Miles, R. (1989) *Racism.* London: Routledge.

Monks, J. (1999) 'It works both ways': belonging and social participation among women with disabilities, in N. Yuval-Davis and P. Werbner (eds) *Women, Citizenship and Difference.* London: Zed Books.

Mooney, G. (1998) 'Remoralizing' the poor? Gender, class and philanthropy in Victorian Britain, in G. Lewis (ed.) *Forming Nation, Framing Welfare.* London: Routledge.

Morris, J. (ed.) (1989) *Able Lives: Women's Experience of Paralysis.* London: The Women's Press.

Morris, J. (1991) *Pride against Prejudice: Transforming Attitudes to Disability.* London: The Women's Press.

Morris, J. (1993a) Prejudice, in J. Swain, V. Finkelstein, S. French and M. Oliver (eds) *Disabling Barriers – Enabling Environments.* London: Sage.

Morris, J. (1993b) *Independent Lives? Community Care and Disabled People.* London: Macmillan.

Morris, J. (ed.) (1996) *Encounters with Strangers: Feminism and Disability.* London: The Women's Press.

Morris, J. (1997) *Community Care: Working in Partnership with Service Users.* Birmingham: Venture Press.

Morris, J. (1998) Creating a space for absent voices: women's experience of receiving assistance with daily living activities, in M. Allott and R. Robb (eds) *Understanding Health and Social Care: An Introductory Reader.* London: Sage.

Morrison, E. and Finkelstein, V. (1993) Broken arts and cultural repair, in J. Swain, V. Finkelstein, S. French and M. Oliver (eds) *Disabling Barriers – Enabling Environments.* London: Sage.

Napolitano, S. (1992) *A Dangerous Woman.* Manchester: Greater Manchester Coalition of Disabled People.

Nettleton, S. (1995) *The Sociology of Health and Illness.* Cambridge: Polity Press.

Nettleton, S. (1998) Health policy, in N. Ellison and C. Pierson (eds) *Developments in British Social Policy.* London: Macmillan.

Nicolaisen, I. (1995) Persons and non-persons: disability and personhood among the Punan Bah of Central Borneo, in B. Ingstad and S. Reynolds Whyte (eds) *Disability and Culture.* Los Angeles: University of California Press.

Nolan, P. (1993) *A History of Mental Health Nursing.* Cheltenham: Stanley Thornes.

Norwich, B. (2000) Brahm Norwich, in P. Clough and J. Corbett (eds) *Theories of Inclusive Education: A Students' Guide.* London: Paul Chapman.

Oliver, M. (1984) The integration and segregation debate: some sociological considerations, *British Journal of Sociology of Education,* 6: 75–92.

Oliver, M. (1988) No place for the voluntaries, *Social Work Today,* 24 November: 10.

Oliver, M. (1990) *The Politics of Disablement.* London: Macmillan.

Oliver, M. (1993) Disability and dependency: a creation of industrial societies, in J. Swain, V. Finkelstein, S. French and M. Oliver (eds) *Disabling Barriers – Enabling Environments.* London: Sage.

Oliver, M. (1996a) A sociology of disability or a disablist sociology?, in L. Barton (ed.) *Disability and Society: Emerging Issues and Insights.* London: Longman.

Oliver, M. (1996b) *Understanding Disability: From Theory to Practice.* London: Macmillan.

Oliver, M. (1999) Final accounts and the parasite people, in M. Corker and S. French (eds) *Disability Discourse.* Buckingham: Open University Press.

Oliver, M. (2001) Disability issues in the postmodern world, in L. Barton (ed.) *Disability Politics and the Struggle for Change.* London: David Fulton.

Oliver, M. and Barnes, C. (1998) *Disabled People and Social Policy: From Exclusion to Inclusion.* London: Longman.

Oliver, M. and Sapey, B. (1999) *Social Work with Disabled People,* 2nd edn. London: Basingstoke: Macmillan.

Oliver, M. and Zarb, G. (1997) The politics of disability: a new approach, in L. Barton and M. Oliver (eds) *Disability Studies: Past, Present and Future.* Leeds: The Disability Press.

Oliver, M., Zarb, G., Silver, J., Moore, M. and Salisbury, V. (1988) *Walking into Darkness: The Experience of Spinal Cord Injury*. London: Macmillan.

Omansky Gordon, B. and Rosenblum, K.E. (2001) Bringing disability into the sociological frame: a comparison of disability with race, sex, and sexual orientation statuses, *Disability and Society*, 16(1): 5–19.

Open University, The (1999) *Understanding Health and Social Care*, OU course K100, Audio 2, side 2. Milton Keynes: The Open University.

Open University, The (2002) *Care, Welfare and Community*, OU course K202, Video 2, programme 2 'Advocacy'. Milton Keynes: The Open University.

Palmer, N., Peacock, C., Turner, F., Vasey, B., supported by Williams, V. (1999) Telling people what you think, in J. Swain and S. French (eds) *Therapy and Learning Difficulties: Advocacy, Participation and Partnership*. Oxford: Butterworth-Heinemann.

Parens, E. and Asch, A. (eds) (2000) *Prenatal Testing and Disability Rights*. Washington, DC: Georgetown University Press.

Park, D.C. and Radford, J.P. (1999) From the case files: restructuring a history of involuntary sterilisation, *Disability and Society*, 13(3): 317–42.

Parker, G. (1993) *With This Body: Caring and Disability in Marriage*. Buckingham: Open University Press.

Parker, M. and Wilson, G. (2000) Diseases of poverty, in T. Alan and A. Thomas (eds) *Poverty and Development: Into the 21st Century*. Oxford: Oxford University Press.

Parr, S., Pound, C., Byng, S. and Long, B. (1999) *The Aphasia Handbook*. York: Joseph Rowntree Foundation.

Paterson, K. and Hughes, B. (1999) Disability studies and phenomenology: the carnal politics of everyday life, *Disability and Society*, 14(5): 597–610.

Paterson, K. and Hughes, B. (2000) Disabled bodies, in P. Handcock, B. Hughes, E. Jagger et al. (eds) *The Body, Culture and Society: An Introduction*. Buckingham: Open University Press.

Payne, G. (2000) An introduction to social division, in G. Payne (ed.) *Social Divisions*. London: Macmillan.

Peace, S. (1998) Caring in place, in A. Brechin, J. Walmsley, J. Katz and S. Peace (eds) *Care Matters: Concepts, Practice and Research in Health and Social Care*. London: Sage.

Pearson, R. (2000) Rethinking gender issues in development, in T. Alan and A. Thomas (eds) *Poverty and Development: Into the 21st Century*. Oxford: Oxford University Press.

Percy-Smith, J. (2000) Introduction: the contours of social exclusion, in J. Percy-Smith (ed.) *Policy Responses to Social Exclusion: Towards Inclusion?* Buckingham: Open University Press.

Pfeiffer, D. and Yoshida, Y. (1995) Teaching disability studies in Canada and the USA, *Disability and Society*, 10(4): 475–500.

Picking, C. (2000) Working in partnership with disabled people: new perspectives for professionals within the social model of disability, in J. Cooper (ed.) *Law, Rights and Disability*. London: Jessica Kingsley.

Potter, D. (2000) The power of colonial states, in T. Alan and A. Thomas (eds) *Poverty and Development: Into the 21st Century*. Oxford: Oxford University Press.

Potts, M. and Fido, R. (1991) *'A Fit Person to be Removed': Personal Accounts of Life in a Mental Deficiency Institution*. Plymouth: Northcote House.

Priestley, M. (1999) *Disability Politics and Community Care*. London: Jessica Kingsley.

Priestley, M. (2001) Introduction: the global context of disability, in M. Priestley (ed.) *Disability and the Life Course: Global Perspectives*. Cambridge: Cambridge University Press.

Rasko, I. and Downes, C. (1995) *Genes in Medicine: Molecular and Human Genetic Disorders*. London: Chapman and Hall.

Reading, P. (1994) *Community Care and the Voluntary Sector*. Birmingham: Venture Press.

Richardson, A. (1989) 'If you love him, let him go', in A. Brechin and J. Walmsley (eds) *Making Connections: Reflecting on the Lives and Experiences of People with Learning Difficulties*. London: Hodder and Stoughton.

Richman, J. (1987) *Medicine and Health*. London: Longman.

Riddell, S. (1996) Theorising special educational needs in a changing political climate, in L. Barton (ed.) *Disability and Society: Emerging Issues and Insights*. London: Longman.

Rioux, M.H. and Bach, M. (eds) (1994) *Disability is Not Measles: New Research Paradigms in Disability*. North York, Ontario: Roeher Institute.

Robb, M. and Davies, C. (1999) Caring communities – fact or fiction?, in *Understanding Health and Social Care* (K100) Open University Course. Milton Keynes: The Open University.

Roberts, K. (2000) Lost in the system: disabled refugees and asylum seekers in Britain, *Disability and Society*, 15(6): 943–8.

Rochester, C. (1995) Voluntary agencies and accountability, in J. Davis Smith, C. Rochester and R. Hedley (eds) *An Introduction to the Voluntary Sector*. London: Routledge.

Rogers, L. (1999) Disabled children will be a 'sin', says scientist, *Sunday Times*, 4 July.

Roulstone, A. (2000) Disability, dependency and the New Deal for disabled people, *Disability and Society*, 15(3): 427–44.

Royal Association for Disability and Rehabilitation (RADAR) (1999) *Genes Are Us? Attitudes to Genetics and Disability: A RADAR survey*. London: RADAR.

Royal Association for Disability and Rehabilitation (RADAR) (2000) *The Human Rights Act 1998: An Overview*. London: RADAR.

Russell, M. (1998) *Beyond Ramps: Disability at the End of the Social Contract*. Monroe, ME: Common Courage Press.

Ryan, J. and Thomas, F. (1987) *The Politics of Mental Handicap*. London: Free Press.

Ryan, T. and Holman, A. (1998) *Able and Willing: Supporting People with Learning Difficulties to Use Direct Payments*. London: Values into Action.

Safer, J. (1996) *Beyond Motherhood: Choosing a Life without Children*. New York: Pocket Books.

Saraga, E. (ed.) (1998) *Embodying the Social: Constructions of Difference*. London: Routledge.

Sattaur, O. (ed.) (2001) *Poverty: Bridging the Gap*. London: Department of International Development.

Schriner, K. (2001) A disability studies perspective on employment issues and policies for disabled people, in G.L. Albrecht, K.D. Seelman and M. Bury (eds) *Handbook of Disability Studies*. London: Sage.

Scotch, R.K. (2001) American disability policy in the twentieth century, in P.K. Longmore and L. Umanski (eds) *The New Disability History: American Perspectives*. New York: New York University Press.

Shakespeare, T. (1996) Disability, identity, difference, in C. Barnes and G. Mercer (eds) *Exploring the Divide: Illness and Disability*. Leeds: The Disability Press.

Shakespeare, T. (1999) Losing the plot? Discourses of disability and genetics, *Sociology of Health and Illness*, 21(5): 669–88.

Shakespeare, T. (2000) *Help: Imagining Welfare*. Birmingham: Venture Press.

Shakespeare, T., Gillespie-Sells, K. and Davies, D. (1996) *The Sexual Politics of Disability: Untold Desires*. London: Cassell.

Shilling, C. (1993) *The Body and Social Theory*. London: Sage.

Silver, L.M. (1998) *Remaking Eden: Cloning and Beyond in a Brave New World*. London: Weidenfeld and Nicolson.

Singer, P. (1979) *Practical Ethics.* New York: Cambridge University Press.

Smith, A. (1994) A damaging experience: black disabled children and their educational and social service provision, in N. Begum, M. Hill and A. Stevens (eds) *Reflections: Views of Black Disabled People on their Lives and Community Care.* London: Central Council for Education and Training in Social Work.

Smith, R. (1996) Sexual constructions and lesbian identity, in T. Cosslet, A. Easton and P. Summerfield (eds) *Women, Power and Resistance: An Introduction to Women's Studies.* Buckingham: Open University Press.

Social Exclusion Unit (1997) *Social Exclusion Unit: Purpose, Work Priorities and Working Methods.* London: HMSO.

Southampton Centre for Independent Living (SCIL) (2000) *A Brief Introduction.* Southampton: SCIL.

Stanton, I. (1996) *Tragic But Brave, Rolling Thunder (CD).* London: Stream Records.

Stone, E. (1999a) Modern slogan, ancient script: impairment and disability in the Chinese language, in M. Corker and S. French (eds) *Disability Discourse.* Buckingham: Open University Press.

Stone, E. (1999b) Disability and development in the majority world, in E. Stone (ed.) *Disability and Development: Learning from Action and Research in the Majority World.* Leeds: The Disability Press.

Stone, E. (2001) A complicated struggle: disability, survival and social change in the majority world, in M. Priestley (ed.) *Disability and the Life Course: Global Perspectives.* Cambridge: Cambridge University Press.

Stone, R. (2000) *Textbook on Civil Liberties and Human Rights,* 3rd edn. London: Blackstone Press.

Stuart, O. (1993) Double oppression: an appropriate starting point?, in J. Swain, V. Finkelstein, S. French and M. Oliver (eds) *Disabling Barriers – Enabling Environments.* London: Sage.

Sutherland, A.T. (1981) *Disabled We Stand.* London: Souvenir Press.

Swain, J. and Cook, T. (2001) In the name of inclusion: 'we all, at the end of the day, have the needs of the children at heart', *Critical Social Policy,* 21(2): 185–208.

Swain, J. and French, S. (1998) Normality and disabling care, in A. Brechin, J. Katz, J. Walmsley and S. Peace (eds) *Care Matters: Concepts, Practice and Research.* London: Sage.

Swain, J. and French, S. (2000) Towards an affirmation model of disability, *Disability and Society,* 15(4): 569–82.

Swain, J. and Lawrence, P. (1994) Learning about disability: changing attitudes or changing understanding?, in S. French (ed.) *On Equal Terms: Working with Disabled People.* Oxford: Butterworth-Heinemann.

Swain, J., Gillman, M. and French, S. (1998) *Confronting Disabling Barriers: Towards Making Organisations Accessible.* Birmingham: Venture Press.

Swain, J., Gillman, M. and Heyman, B. (1999) Challenging questions, in J. Swain and S. French (eds) *Therapy and Learning Difficulties: Advocacy, Participation and Partnership.* Oxford: Butterworth-Heinemann.

Tarrow, S. (1998) *Power in Movement: Social Movements, Collective Action and Politics,* 2nd edn. Cambridge: Cambridge University Press.

Tarver, M.A., Benson, S. and Thomas, C. (1993) Therapists' approaches to the emotional needs of their patients. Paper presented at the Mental Health Needs of Disabled People Conference, Douglas Bader Centre, Queen Mary's University Hospital, Roehampton, 3rd March.

Thomas, A. (1992) Non-governmental organisations and the limits to empowerment, in M. Whyte, M. Mackintosh and T. Hewitt (eds) *Development, Poverty and Public Action.* Oxford: Oxford University Press.

Thomas, A. (2000) Meanings and views of development, in T. Allen and A. Thomas (eds) *Poverty and Development: Into the 21st Century*. Oxford: Oxford University Press.

Thomas, A. and Allen, T. (2000) Agencies of development, in T. Allen and A. Thomas (eds) *Poverty and Development: Into the 21st Century*. Oxford: Oxford University Press.

Thomas, C. (1999) *Female Forms: Experiencing and Understanding Disability*. Buckingham: Open University Press.

Thomas, G., Walker, D. and Webb, J. (1998) *The Making of the Inclusive School*. London: Routledge.

Thompson, N. (1998) *Promoting Equality: Challenging Discrimination and Oppression in the Human Services*. London: Macmillan.

Thompson, N. (2001) *Anti-Discriminatory Practice*, 3rd edn. Basingstoke: Palgrave.

Thomson, R.G. (1997) *Extraordinary Bodies: Figuring Physical Disability in American Culture and Literature*. New York: Columbia University Press.

Toates, F. (1996) The embodied self: a biological perspective, in R. Stevens (ed.) *Understanding the Self*. London: Sage.

Tomlinson, S. (1982) *A Sociology of Special Education*. London: Routledge and Kegan Paul.

Tomlinson, S. and Colquhoun, R.F. (1995) The political economy of special educational needs in Britain, *Disability and Society*, 10(2): 191–202.

Trade Union Disability Alliance (TUDA) (1997) *Why the Disability Discrimination Act Must Be Repealed and Replaced with Civil Rights for Disabled People*. London: TUDA.

Turner, B.S. (1993) Contemporary problems in the theory of citizenship, in B.S. Turner (ed.) *Citizenship and Social Theory*. London: Sage.

Turner, B.S. (1996) *The Body and Society*, 2nd edn. London: Sage.

Turner, B.S. (2001) Disability and the sociology of the body, in G.L. Albrecht, K.D. Seelman and M. Bury (eds) *Handbook of Disability Studies*. London: Sage.

Union of the Physically Impaired Against Segregation (UPIAS) (1976) *Fundamental Principles of Disability*. London: UPIAS.

Vasey, S. (1992a) A response to Liz Crow, *Coalition*, September: 43–4.

Vasey, S. (1992b) Disability culture: it's a way of life, in R. Rieser and M. Mason (eds) *Disability Equality in the Classroom: A Human Rights Issue*. London: Disability Equality in Education.

Vernon, A. (1994) Black and minority ethnic people receive poorer quality social services, in N. Begum, M. Hill and A. Stevens (eds) *Reflections: Views of Black Disabled People on their Lives and Community Care*. London: Central Council for Education and Training in Social Work.

Walmsley, J. (1993) Contradictions in caring; reciprocity and interdependence, *Disability, Handicap and Society*, 8(2): 129–41.

Walmsley, J. (1996) 'Doing what mum wants me to do': looking at family relationships from the point of view of adults with intellectual disabilities, *Journal of Applied Research in Intellectual Disabilities*, 9(4): 324–41.

Ward, A. (1997) Working with young people in residential settings, in J. Roche and S. Tucker (eds) *Youth and Society: Contemporary Theory, Policy and Practice*. London: Sage.

Warnock, H.M. (chairman) (1978) *Special Educational Needs Report of the Enquiry into the Education of Handicapped Children and Young People* (Warnock Report). London: HMSO.

Wates, M. and Jade, R. (1999) *Bigger than the Sky: Disabled Women on Parenting*. London: The Women's Press.

Weale, A. (2001) *Science and the Swastika*. Basingstoke: Channel 4 Books.

Wendell, S. (1996) *The Rejected Body: Feminist Philosophical Perspectives on Disability*. London: Routledge.

Wendell, S. (1997) Towards a feminist theory of disability, in L. Davis (ed.) *The Disability Studies Reader.* London: Routledge.

Westcott, H. and Cross, M. (1996) *This Far and No Further: Towards Ending the Abuse of Disabled Children.* Birmingham: Venture Press.

Williams, F. (1996) Postmodernism, feminism and the question of difference, in N. Parton (ed.) *Social Theory, Social Change and Social Work.* London: Routledge.

Williams, F. (1997) Anthology: care, in J. Bornat, J. Johnson, C. Pereira, D. Pilgrim and F. Williams (eds) *Community Care: A Reader.* London: Macmillan.

Williams, I. (1989) *The Alms Trade: Charities, Past, Present and Future.* London: Routledge and Kegan Paul.

Wilmot, F. and Saul, P. (1998) *A Breath of Fresh Air: Birmingham's Open-Air Schools 1911–1970.* Chichester: Phillimore.

Wirz, S. and Hartley, S. (1999) Challenges for Universities of the north interested in community based rehabilitation, in E. Stone (ed.) *Disability and Development: Learning from Action and Research on Disability in the Majority World.* Leeds: The Disability Press.

Wise, S. (1996) Feminist activism: continuity and change, in T. Cosslett, A. Easton and P. Summerfield (eds) *Women, Power and Resistance: An Introduction to Women's Studies.* Buckingham: Open University Press.

Wolbring, G. (2001) Where do we draw the line? Surviving eugenics in a technological world, in M. Priestley (ed.) *Disability and the Life Course: Global Perspectives.* Cambridge: Cambridge University Press.

Wood, R. (1991) Care of disabled people, in G. Dalley (ed.) *Disability and Social Policy.* London: Policy Studies Institute.

Woodward, K. (2000) Questions of identity, in K. Woodward (ed.) *Questioning Identity: Gender, Class, Nation.* London: Routledge in association with The Open University.

World Health Organization (WHO) (2001) *The World Health Report.* Geneva: WHO.

Young, I.M. (2000) *Inclusion and Democracy.* Oxford: Oxford University Press.

Young, M. and Willmott, P. (1957) *Family and Kinship in East London.* London: Pelican.

Zames Fleischer, D. and Zames, F. (2001) *The Disability Rights Movement: From Charity to Confrontation.* Philadelphia, PA: Temple University Press.

Zorza, R. and Zorza, V. (1993) A way to die, in D. Dickenson and M. Johnson (eds) *Death, Dying and Bereavement.* London: Sage.

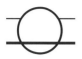

Index

DISABILITY, HUMAN RIGHTS AND EDUCATION
CROSS-CULTURAL PERSPECTIVES

Felicity Armstrong and Len Barton (eds.)

This book recognizes the importance of an informed cross-cultural understanding of the policies and practices of different societies within the field of disability, human rights and education. It represents an attempt to critically engage with issues arising from the historical and contemporary domination of portrayals of 'the western' as advanced, democratic and exemplary, in contrast to the construction of 'the rest of the world' as backward, primitive and inferior in these fundamental areas. How human rights are understood in different contexts is a key theme in this book. Importantly, some contributors raise questions about the value of a 'human rights' model across all societies. Other contributors see the struggle for human rights as at the heart of the struggle for an inclusive society. The implications for education arising from this debate are identified, and a series of questions is raised by each author for further reflection and discussion as well as providing a stimulus for developing future research.

Disability, Human Rights and Education is recommended reading for students and researchers interested in Disability Studies, inclusive education and social policy. It is also directly relevant to professionals and policy makers in the field seeking a greater understanding of cross-cultural perspectives.

Contents
Introduction – Disabled people's quest for social justice in Zimbabwe – Human rights and the struggle for inclusive education in Trinidad and Tobago – Headlights on full beam: disability and education in Hong Kong – Human rights and inclusive education in China: a Western perspective – Rights and disabilities in educational provision in Pakistan and Bangladesh: roots, rhetoric, reality – Inclusive education in Canada: a piece in the equality puzzle – Disability, human rights and education: the United States – Special education and human rights in Australia: how do we know about disablement, and what does it mean for educators? – Educational opportunities and polysemic notions of equality in France – Experience-near perspectives on disabled people's rights in Sweden – Equality and full participation for all? School practices and special education/integration in Greece – Disability, human rights and education in Cyprus – Disability, human rights and education in Romania – 'Is there anyone there concerned with human rights?' Cross-cultural connections, disability and the struggle for change in England – Index.

Contributors
Derrick Armstrong, Felicity Armstrong, Len Barton, Nathalie Bélanger, Robert Chimedza, Karen Dunn, Nicolas Garant, Alan Gartner, Anders Gustavsson, Farhad Hossain, Dorothy Kerzner Lipsky, John Lewis, M. Miles, Michele Moore, Ann Cheryl Namsoo, Susan Peters, Helen Phtiaka, Patricia Potts, Marcia Rioux, Roger Slee, Anastasia Vlachou-Balafouti.

256pp   0 335 20457 0 (Paperback)   0 335 20458 9 (Hardback)

RESEARCHING DISABILITY ISSUES

Michele Moore, Sarah Beazley and June Maelzer

This book is designed to meet a growing need for clear illustrations of how to carry out research which seeks to explore disability issues. It aims to demonstrate the value of a critical attention to social, rather than medical starting points for researching disability, through reviewing a variety of studies which look at different aspects of disabled people's lives. Different quantitative and qualitative methodological frameworks are considered ranging from analysis of observation data concerning disabled children in schools to rich conversation-based data which focuses on family life. A central theme concerns the pivotal role of disabled people in research. The book provides substantive examples of the dilemmas which face researchers and connects these to ideas for individual personal action. Disabled and non-disabled researchers, professionals and students from a wide range of disciplines will find the presentation of both research findings and debates informative and of interest.

Contents

128pp   0 335 19803 1 (Paperback)   0 335 19804 X (Hardback)

DISABILITY, THE FAMILY AND SOCIETY
LISTENING TO MOTHERS

Janet Read

Circumstances dictate that many mothers play a central role in the upbringing of their disabled children. Mothers and children often find themselves involved in an unusually intimate and protracted relationship. This book explores mothers' perspectives about the ways that they find themselves acting as mediators between their children and a world that can be hostile to their interests. It takes as its starting point a study in which mothers from diverse backgrounds detail the ways in which they attempt to represent their children to the world, and the world to their children in both formal and informal interactions. They describe challenging discussions with children and other family members as well as battles and negotiations elsewhere. Their particular experiences and perspectives are linked to wider research and theory on motherhood and caring, the life patterns of disabled children and their families, and the discrimination faced by disabled children and adults.

Disability, the Family and Society will be of interest to students of disability studies, sociology, women's studies, social policy and social and community work.

Contents

156pp   0 335 20310 8 (Paperback)   0 335 20311 6 (Hardback)

FEMALE FORMS
EXPERIENCING AND UNDERSTANDING DISABILITY

Carol Thomas

- What is the relevance of feminist ideas for understanding women's experiences of disability?
- How can the social model of disability be developed theoretically?
- What are the key differences between disability studies and medical sociology?

In answer to these questions, this book explores and develops ideas about disability, engaging with important debates in disability studies about what disability is and how to theorize it. It also examines the interface between disability studies, women's studies and medical sociology, and offers an accessible review of contemporary debates and theoretical approaches. The title *Female Forms* reflects two things about the book: first, its use of disabled women's experiences, as told by themselves, to bring a number of themes to life, and second, the author's belief in the importance of feminist ideas and debates for disability studies. The social model of disability is the book's bedrock, but the author both challenges and contributes to social modelist thought. She advances a materialist feminist perspective on disability, producing a book which is of multi-disciplinary relevance.

Female Forms will be useful to the growing number of students on disability studies courses, as well as those interested in women's studies, medical sociology and social policy. It will also appeal to those studying or working in the health and social care professions such as nursing, social work, occupational therapy and physiotherapy.

Contents

192pp   0 335 19693 4 (Paperback)   0 335 19694 2 (Hardback)

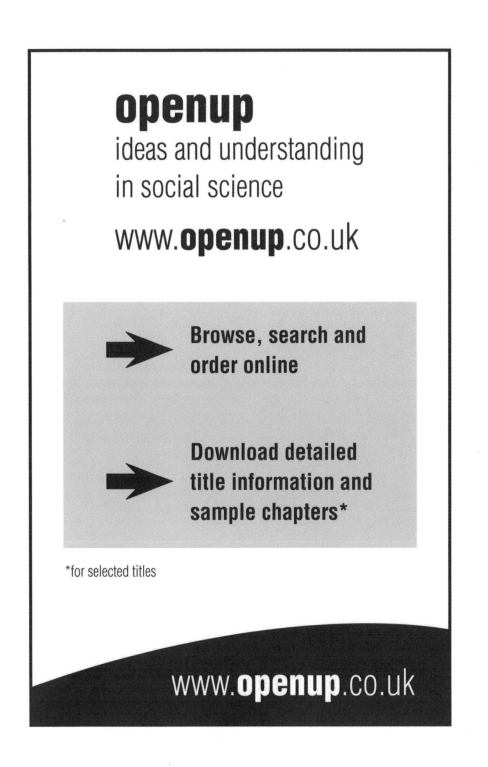